WEIGHT LIFTING FOR WOMEN

A WEIGHT LOSS PROGRAM IN 4 STEPS

Sal J. Marcotte

MEDICAL DISCLAIMER

This book is meant for educational and information purposes only. It is not meant to give any medical advice, diagnose, or treat any medical conditions. No medical claims are made in this book. The nutrition and exercise advice given in this book will not treat or cure medical conditions, metabolic disorders, or other illnesses. The fitness and nutritional advice is meant for healthy individuals who want to improve their appearance for cosmetic reasons and not to treat illnesses of any kind.

You should always consult your physician or other healthcare provider should you have any questions regarding a medical condition or treatment plan.

The author is not a MD or RD and cannot be held liable or responsible to any person or entity with respect to any information contained in this book. The reader/ user assumes all risks for any injury, loss or damage caused or alleged to be caused directly or indirectly by using the information contained in this book.

Table of Contents

Introduction.. 6

Step1: Decoding the Word Nutrition.............. 11

    Macronutrients: The Building Bricks of Your Body... 12

    Micronutrients: Limited but valuable......... 16

    Is drinking more water healthy? Well, it depends... 20

    Food, Glorious Food! 26

    Your Diet Needs Fewer of These................ 28

    Supplements – Just a Hype or Helpful?.... 30

    Nutrition for Sports and Exercise: Boost Your Energy!... 32

    Taking Care of Nutrition during Menopause: 5 Tips Plus 1...37

Step2: Making Way for a Healthier Lifestyle.. 41

    Healthy Habits Lead to a Healthy You 42

    14 Easy Ways to Develop Healthy Habits 47

Step 3: How Our Body Reacts To Training, And More..55

    Know Your Body Type and Optimize Your Lifestyle 56

    How to Train the Right Way as Per Your Body Somatotype 62

How Fat Burns Inside Your Body 64

Discover How Muscles React to Training 66

Weights Would Make You Look Muscly... And Other False Myths! 69

Exercising During Periods: What a Great Idea! 75

Exercising During Pregnancy? With The Right Precautions... 79

Exercising During Menopause? It's a Must! 84

Step 4: Design your Own Workout Session and Become your Own Trainer 90

Cardio or Strength Training: Which is Better? 92

First Time at the Gym? Some Tips and Slangs... 99

Equipment, Machines and Accessories: How to Use Those Strange Objects without an Engineering Degree! 104

Stretching Exercises to Master 116

Weight Loss Program 123

Conclusion 160

Introduction

Staying healthy was never easy. Weight lifting is out of option.Losing weight is a task next to impossible for a lot of women. And this is because, more often than not, they hardly get time for themselves. No, I will not blame them for their messed-up lifestyle...

Most of the time, they are busy taking care of their kids, cooking for their husband, washing dishes, taking care of the home, and managing their professional lives.

Sad but the truth.

All these tasks are important, and may have a deeper meaning in their life. Yes, there are a lot of women who are HAPPY and SATISFIED with the way they are.

But you will agree with me that every woman deserves to stay healthy. These are things that your body might be signaling you about - might be approaching menopause, you might be pregnant or you might be facing difficulties in conceiving, your body might be feeling tired due to exhaustive list of things that you take care of, you might need rest, you might be deficient in certain vitamins, and the list is endless. Identify these signs and make a plan to deal with them.

This is why I am here with this book in which I will teach you how to lose weight and lift weights without introducing a hell lot of changes in your routine.

No pictures "before" and "after" (you are you, and no one else) and no promises, no motivational phrases "you can do it". If you're reading this book, you know it depends on you.

Usually, the books easily available are of 300-400 pages consisting of detailed descriptions of exercises, with seductive pictures of models with unreachable bodies... but you –the reader - have no time to lose and you are an intelligent woman.

If you have free time and you are looking for books on the subject, it's because you want an agile booklet with simple notions, useful and easy-to-apply tips to get back in shape. A personal coach that takes you by hand and provide you with a step by step guide to a healthier lifestyle. Isn't it?

This is a small but comprehensive guide to the topic of fitness and it aims to provide you with a guide to nutrition and the correct lifestyle because these are essential elements - together with the right dose of exercise (read: stretching, weight lifting, and the like) -to quickly gain an enviable physical form that lasts over time.

Well, I do not want to waste your time: if you prefer to jump directly to the exercises, go to Step4. But on doing this, you will end up missing the most important part – preparing your body to make the most out of the exercises. Don't say that I didn't warn you earlier *wink*.

Oh yes, I forgot, here are a few a disclaimers that I want to make:

- No, this guide is not a magic potion. It will NOT provide you with baseless claims and methods and promise you to make healthy within a span of weeks or so.
- No, this guide doesn't contain random before and after pictures. Neither will this book make any promises, and motivational phrases without any solid info.
- No, this guide doesn't contain countless pages with tough-to-follow exercises and postures with seductive pictures which shame your body instead of inspiring you.

So what is this book all about?

- This book respects you as a woman, an intelligent woman, and understands that you have a tough routine to meet. You have loving kids, an understanding partner, and a little time for yourself.
- This book respects your choices as a woman, and respects that you hardly get any time for exercising all because of the varied jobs that you are expected to accomplish, both in personal and professional front.
- This book guides you and walks with you to help you lead a healthier life in an easy-to-follow format.
- This book is a handy personal coach which provides you with actionable insights on how you can eat well, sleep tight, and get a better shape without making your life turn upside down.
- This book introduces you to the world of exercises, their types, the technical jargons, and everything in between.

All in all, this book focuses on a deeper picture. Let's face it, staying healthy is not just about exercising. It is a bigger concept, and has a deeper meaning attached to it.

Speaking from personal experience, as an experienced personal trainer and gym instructor, I have seen people hitting the gym, exercising for a while, and having coke along with French fries soon after. Will this lead to a healthier lifestyle? Definitely, no!

Staying healthy is a cumulative effort wherein you understand the requirements of your body and fulfill them holistically. Thus, this book is a lot more than a simple 45-minute workout plan. This is a small yet comprehensive guide which tells you how to lead your lifestyle healthily, no matter how much busy you are.

Here is a final call for all the women out there – start taking care of your health before it becomes too late!

Get started and explore what makes this book different than thousands of others available in the market.

Step1: Decoding the Word Nutrition

Nutrition, nourishment or aliment – whatever you term it, undoubtedly plays an important role in our overall well-being. Generally speaking, it is the supply of food to provide proper energy to our body to keep it functioning properly.

Here are some quick facts on nutrition which you must know about:

- Our body requires seven major kinds of nutrients to stay healthy.
- Although required in smaller amounts, micronutrients play an important role in our body.
- Vitamins are important, but our body cannot synthesize them.
- Nutrients play an important role in our body, but not all of them provide us with energy, such as fiber and water.

This sounds interesting, right? Sure, it does. But believe me, nutrition is a tough nut to crack. And I realized this after having a talk with a girl in the gym I used to do cardio in. Quite appalled and confused with what her dietitian recommended her, one day she couldn't stop herself and asked her dietitian – why dietary advice is so confusing?

Although I didn't follow her conversation with the dietitian (good manners, you see?), her question actually hit me hard. There is quite a chaos when it comes to nutrition. Nuts, for instance, were considered too fatty to eat in large amount, are now considered healthy. Eggs, once believed to have too much cholesterol, are back in the healthy-foods list.

So what is this all about? As expected, the answers to all your dietary questions, and the reasons behind why your dietitian wants you to consume certain things and skip the rest depend on macronutrients, micronutrients, and minerals that you consume. Let's know more about them in detail.

Macronutrients: The Building Bricks of Your Body

If you are a fitness enthusiast and like to keep yourself updated with the fitness industry every now and then, I'm sure you must have heard about macros. What exactly are they?

Confused?

Well, as the name suggests, macros or macronutrients are nutritional compounds that your body needs in significant amountsfor proper functioning. Majorly, they can be classified as proteins, fats, and carbohydrates. Each of these plays an important role in our bodies. Let's find out more about them.

Carbohydrates

Consisting of starch and sugar, carbohydrates are one of the macronutrients that our body needs the most. This is because our body breaks down most carbs easily to release energy in the form of glucose.Glucose, after getting released, enters our cells to trigger a series of metabolic reactions which convert the glucose into Adenosine Tri-Phosphate (do not Google! This is a form of cellular energy).

All the glucose which remains unused is converted into starch and is stored in our liver as glycogen to be used by the body later on.

As a matter of fact, if you are not on a diet plan (like the intermittent fasting), carbohydrates must make up around 50% of your energy needs, but the exact amount depends on your body-type. I will talk about this in the later sections of this book.

Protein

Known as the building blocks of the body, proteins comprise of twenty different types of amino acids. Amino acids are used by our body in three different ways – as a building material, as an energy source, as a building block for building new proteins for proper cellular functioning.

Out of the twenty types of amino acids, nine of these are categorized into essential amino acids. This means that your body can't meet the needs of these acids internally, and thus, you are required to consume them through food. The other eleven can either be produced by the liver or they can be consumed through diet.

It is important to mention here that proteins are vital for varied kinds of needs – for the proper functioning of our organs, for luscious hair, for strong and shiny nails, and for other important purposes. Thus, if you want to improve the quality of your hair and nails, you know what to consume!

Fats

You might regard fats as your biggest enemy, most women do! Quite differentfrom what you might have learned and heard, fats play an important role in the functioning of our body. We need them to stay healthy. In fact, 20-30% of our food should consist of fats, depending on your body type.

What make fats a bit harmful to our body are their high-calorie levels. Contrary to proteins and carbohydrates which contain four calories per gram, fats contain nine calories per gram which makes them a bit problematic.

Nevertheless, proteins still play an important role in keeping our bodies healthy, regulating our hormones, and keeping our nerves in a top-notch condition.

What's more, fats also act as a storehouse of energy. Our body uses them for storing unused calories. You might argue that unused calories are stored as glucose. Sure, they are. But that's just a small amount. On the other hand, fats enable our body to store unlimited amounts of energy which can then be brought to use while exercising, sleeping, and performing other such activities.

Fats can be further subdivided into three categories:

- Trans fat: This is the type of fat you must stay away from. It is found in snacks, fast food, and the likes.
- Saturated fat: This is generally obtained from butter, cream, meat, and other animal sources.
- Unsaturated fat: This is procured from plant sources like olive oil, canola oil, nuts and the like.

Micronutrients: Limited but valuable

Think of vitamins and minerals – these are nothing but micronutrients. Similar to macronutrients, our body needs micronutrients to be able to function properly. However, unlike macronutrients, micronutrients are not required in large amounts, instead, just minuscule amount of them is enough for our body to stay healthy.

Although needed in small amount, they have a vital role to play. Deficiency of any of the vitamins and minerals can lead to deficiencies which can have an everlasting and detrimental effect on our health.

Vitamins

Vitamins, a kind of micronutrient, are needed in small amounts. Almost all the vitamins are obtained from external sources except for Vitamin D. Let's know more about each of the vitamins in detail.

Fat Soluble Vitamins

These are the kind of vitamins that can be stored in fatty tissues for future use. To ensure proper absorption of these fats, it is highly recommended to consume them along with healthy fats.

- Vitamin A

Essential for brain and eye health, vitamin A is an essential vitamin for our immune system. Vitamin A can be easily obtained from both plant and animal sources. However, it is highly recommended to consume it only from the plant sources to rule out any chances of toxicity.

- Vitamin D

Vitamin D functions both as a micronutrient and a hormone and plays a vital role in maintaining our bone health. Additionally, it also keeps our respiratory system healthy and takes care of our emotional and mental well-being.

- Vitamin E

Also knows as powerhouse antioxidant, vitamin E is known for its anti-oxidant properties. This vitamin protects oxidation of delicate lipids. Additionally, vitamin E has another important role to play. It takes care of your DNA by fighting against free radicals, thus preventing them from modifying the structure of your chromosomes.

- Vitamin K

Vitamin K ensures that there are enough proteins in the blood to ensure proper clotting, whenever required.

Water Soluble Vitamins

As the name suggests, water-soluble vitamins are soluble in water. This is the reason why they are often expelled out of our body through urine. This is why you must replace them on a daily basis as they cannot be stored in our bodies.

- Vitamins B-Complex

The B-complex vitamins consist of a group of vitamins including riboflavin (B2), pantothenic acid (B5), cobalamin (B12), folic acid (B9), niacin (B3), thiamin (B1), and pyridoxine(B6). These vitamins, like others, also play an active role in our body. They regulate the release of energy in our cells and also impact our immune health and mood.

Vitamin B9 and B12 have an even important role to play. They take care of our brain health and preserve our memory and cognitive abilities as we age.

- Vitamin C

Often found in moisturizers, and other skin care products, Vitamin C is perhaps the best vitamin of all the beauty brands out there. This is because it is an antioxidant and takes care of our skin, and bones.

Minerals

Similar to vitamins, minerals are also an essential micronutrient. They are organic substances and occur naturally. Minerals can be divided into two: macrominerals and trace minerals. As you might predict, our body needs macrominerals in larger amounts when compared to trace minerals.

<u>Macrominerals</u>

These include sodium, potassium, chlorine, phosphorous and the likes.

- Magnesium

Important for our bone health, magnesium plays a vital role in our body metabolism and also acts as a cofactor in various chemical reactions in our body.

- Calcium

You must have often heard about the importance of calcium in determining the strength of our body. But calcium not only keeps our bones strong, but it also plays an important role in the successful relaxation and contraction of our muscles and other related tasks.

- Potassium

This is one mineral you might be lacking on. Most Americans do, approximately 98%, primarily due to inadequate plant food intake! Responsible for cell detoxification, and proper functioning of our nerves and muscles, potassium intake is important for our body.

<u>Trace minerals</u>

As already discussed, our body needs trace minerals in much lesser amount when compared to macrominerals. While macrominerals must be consumed in grams, trace minerals must only be consumed in milligrams(1/1,000 of a gram) and even micrograms(1/1,000,000 of a gram). Some of the top trace minerals that our body needs include iodine, chromium, zinc, copper, iron and the like.

Is drinking morewater healthy? Well, it depends...

As is evident, our body needs macronutrients and micronutrients, all because of the different role that each of them plays. However, that's not just it.

Water also plays an important role in our body and this is why it is recommended to drink around 6 to 8, 8-ounce glasses of water each day. Sounds reasonable, right?

But here is the catch – not all of us require the same quantity of water to stay hydrated. While some people feel thirsty every thirty minutes, there are others who stay healthy even after drinking fewer than 8 glasses of water each day.

The best indicator if you are drinking enough water is to check your urine. If it is amber color or dark yellow, the chances are high that you may be dehydrated. On the other hand, if it is light yellow or almost colorless, you are doing just fine!

It is worth mentioning here that you don't have to only drink water to stay hydrated. Consuming fresh juices milk, herbal teas, and other similar beverages can also keep you hydrated.

Finding it difficult to stay hydrated? Here are a few tips which might come to your rescue:

- Carry a water bottle with you wherever you go. The chances are high that you will end up drinking water whenever you will feel bored.
- If plain water doesn't suit your taste buds, you can try adding a slice of lime or lemon to your drink
- If you often forget drinking water, it is the best practice to develop a schedule. Drink water on waking up, after having breakfast, while watching TV, and so on.
- Make sure that you drink water before and after a workout.
- You can even drink water when you feel hungry. This will help you in surpassing hunger, and will keep your body in shape!

How will you know if you are dehydrated? Here are a few pointers:

- Dry mouth
- Thirst

- Confusion
- No tears when you cry
- Dizziness
- No urine, or little urine
- Dark colored urine
- Headache

Stay away from these symptoms by taking care of your water intake from day 1. You might be at a higher risk of dehydration if you have a certain medical condition like an infection in the bladder, stones in the kidney or if you are sick or pregnant or breastfeeding.

This brings us to an important question, what should you drink and what you should not?

Let's find out.

Drink: What is Recommended and What is Not?

- Drink semi-skimmed, 1% fat or skimmed milk

Milk is the supreme source of calcium, a mineral which is responsible for making the bones stronger and healthier. It also contains various vitamins, proteins, and minerals which prevent our teeth from any kind of decay.

However, it is important to mention here that not all types of milk contain the same levels of vitamins and minerals. Some of them are rich in minerals and proteins and some are rich in low fat. The healthier choices when it comes to milk include drinking either semi-skimmed, 1% fat or skimmed milk.

Skimmed milk is low in fat and high on calcium. 1% fat milk also has a lower content of fat along with some of the essential proteins. Avoid drinking sugar-rich drinks like milkshakes, milk-based energy drinks, condensed milk and such.

- Juices, and smoothies

Fruits juices and smoothies are mouthwatering, especially in summers. But you need to stop having a sweet tooth to remain healthy. Though they contain a variety of minerals which are beneficial for your health, eating the fruit is recommended.

Even the 100% unsweetened fruit juices, vegetable juices are not healthy. For instance, drinking 2 glasses of fruit juice or smoothie will only count as 1 portion. This is because juices and smoothies lack the fiber content in them which can only be consumed in a large amount when you eat whole fruits and vegetables.

On top of that, fruit juices and smoothies have high sugar content. However, drinking fruits along with your meal is better.

Your total intake of the fruit juice, vegetable juice, and smoothies in a day should not exceed 150ml which amounts to nearly a small glass.

- Fizzy drinks, flavored water, and squashes with added sugar

Fizzy drink, flavored water, and squashes have the lowest content of nutrients in them and should, therefore, be avoided. Plus they contain sugar to a level which is unhealthy. So always check the calorie content in them before buying. High sugar content and high-calorie content make you gain weight and should, therefore, be avoided.

- Tea and coffee

The two common caffeinated drinks are tea and coffee. It is fine to consume tea and coffee in medium quantity as part of your daily routine until it is not in excess. Caffeinated drinks make you pee more often. So, if you have a urine continence problem, drinking tea and coffee is not recommended. However, trying alternative drinks and drinking low caffeinated tea and coffee are allowed.

Also, if you want to cut sweetness out of your drinks, you can choose the artificial sweetness to lower the sugar content. They are really helpful if you want to cut down on your sugar intake level.

- Energy drinks and caffeine

Energy drinks are rich in caffeine and sugar. These drinks also contain stimulants and some amount of vitamins and minerals, if you are lucky enough.

One small can of around 250ml of energy drink contains 80mg of caffeine which is equivalent to drinking a mug of coffee. If you are drinking thinking they are healthier, I am sorry – they are not.

- Sports drinks

Sports drinks are drinks that are consumed when you are involved in high-level sports activities. Such drinks are known to boost your energy while on the ground.

Though meant to increase your energy, these drinks also have a high content of sugar and caffeine in them. The only liquid that you need to drink while involved in a sports activity is water. Water is the healthier fluid and won't harm your body in any way.

- Soda

Soda has no nutritional value and is completely useless to drink if you are drinking it for health purposes. Carbonated soda should be avoided in all respects. It increases the chances of being diabetic, has no nutrients in them, makes you gain weight, has high sugar content and also contains phosphoric acid. It also leads to dehydration and can damage your teeth.

I don't think you need any other better reason to avoid soda if you want to live a healthier life. Drink soda once in a blue moon to satisfy your taste bud.

More than half of the juices and drinks are just dissolved sugar and caffeine that should not be consumed in high quantities if you are taking a step ahead towards living a healthier life.

Food, Glorious Food!

Whatever you eat throughout the day, every single meal that you consume is important and plays an active role in helping you lead a healthier lifestyle. Thus, it is essential that you watch out what you eat, how much you eat, and when you eat.

Here is what you must include in your meal if you want to build muscles and lose weight:

- Whole grains

Try hard to ensure that at least half of your grains are whole grains. While shopping grocery, look for the label *100% whole grain* or *100% whole wheat* to be on a safer side. Why all the fuss related to whole grains, you ask? This is because whole grains provide more nutrients when compared to their refined counterparts.

- Veggies and fruits

Needless to say, you must consume both vegetables and fruits for good health. While buying fruits, make sure that you have enough of red and orange color, on the other hand, while buying vegetables, focus on the green.

- Dairy

No meal is complete without a cup of low-fat or fat-free milk. Both fat-free and low-fat milk provide you with the same amount of calcium as is provided with whole milk but fewer calories. Can't stand milk? How about trying soymilk or even low-fat yogurt? Explore your options.

- Lean protein

Including foods rich in protein is a must. It is highly recommended to include foods like beans, pork, chicken, lean beef, tofu, turkey, eggs and the like to meet your daily protein requirements.

- Soybeans

If you often have heavier periods and tend to lose a lot of blood during menstruation, soybeans can prove to be highly advantageous. Soybeans are a good source of vitamin K, iron, and phosphorous along with proteins.

- Protein powders

If you want to build muscles, protein powders can prove to be helpful. Although you can choose to get protein from foods alone, if you are somehow struggling to meet your daily requirements, you can choose to go for protein shakes.

However, it is important to keep in mind that you must choose protein powders meant for women. Although protein is protein, but the protein powders meant for women also contain a range of ingredients that plays a vital role in a woman's body like Vitamin B6, iron, and Folic Acid.

- Nuts and seeds

Nuts and seeds like peanuts, flax seeds, and sunflower seeds are a great source of minerals, healthy fats, proteins, vitamins and fibers. Almonds, for instance, are a great source of vitamin E, phosphorous, and magnesium.

- Brown rice

Brown rice is not a great source of protein, but they do contain carbohydrates which fuel you to perform physical activities effortlessly. Thus, if you are going to perform an intensive workout or exercise, consuming brown rice a few hours before the practice session could be a great idea.

Your Diet Needs Fewer of These

Not everything edible is worth eating and consuming. There are certain foods which must be avoided, no matter what:

- Alcohol

Needless to say, alcohol is a strong deterrent to your normal well-being. It impacts your body muscles adversely and can even impact your liver.

- Added sugars

Foods rich in sugar must be avoided. Whether it is a sports drink or soda, or candy, ice cream, cake, and cookies – all of them contain added sugars which are high on calories.

- Deep-fried foods

Deep-fried foods promote inflammation and can make you prone to various diseases. While you can consume onion rings, fried fish, and French fries once in a while, you must avoid them as much as possible. As a matter of fact, deep-fried foods also work against your objective of losing weight.

- Junk food

Although heavenly in taste, junk foods are not good for your overall health, all because they contain a lot many calories, generally in the form of fat and sugar. This means that you do not get any fiber, minerals or vitamins from them, but just calories. Some foods that fall under this category and must not be a part of your diet include pastries, soda, candy, cookies, soda, chips and the like.

- Frozen products

Frozen foods are a bit no, all because they contain a large number of preservatives, and high levels of sodium in them which is not healthy at all.

- Bottled smoothies

Bottled smoothies are an important part of the breakfast for most of us, but this timesaving drink has its own drawback: it is high in calories and sugar and must not be in your to-eat list, especially if you want to keep your waistline slim.

- Salt

You might not see this coming but it is highly recommended to reduce your salt intake. This is because table salt contains sodium chloride. Excessive levels of sodium in your diet can lead to problems related to blood pressure and might also put you at risk of heart stroke.

- Saturated and trans fat

Although both saturated and trans fat are edible, they are found to impact your coronary artery adversely. They work by raising levels of bad cholesterol and reducing the levels of good cholesterol in your blood.

These were just a few of the many items that must be avoided at all costs.

Supplements – Just a Hype or Helpful?

Visit a grocery store, and you will come across towering shelves of vitamin and mineral supplements and even taller claims claiming that supplements are what your body needs.

All this sounds lucrative especially when just taking care of your health seems to be as simple as swallowing a pill. But are these claims true, and are supplements really helpful?

Well, before you start consuming all the minerals and vitamins right from vitamin A to zinc, it is essential to keep in mind that nothing can benefit you more than having a balanced diet consisting of healthy foods.

Focus on Food

Most nutritionists recommend consuming foods and having a wholesome meal consisting of a range of foods with a variety of minerals and vitamins to meet your body's nutritional needs naturally. Although supplements might provide your body with the required chemical formula, they will fail to meet the dietary fiber requirements of your body. What's more, if you consume fat-soluble vitamins on an empty stomach without any food, the essential nutrients will not be absorbed well by your body.

Supplements are secondary

Although having a balanced diet is important, supplements could prove to be helpful. This is because no matter how balanced diet you try to have, your diet might still be deficient in some areas. This is where supplements can help.

However, it is important to note that you must use supplements as a supplement and not as a replacementfor your food. You should only take those supplements which are recommended by your healthcare professional.

Nutrition forSports and Exercise: Boost Your Energy!

Proper nutrition is necessary to ensure that your body functions properly. Nutrition for exercise can be divided into three parts:

- Before the exercise
- During the exercise
- After the exercise

Before The Exercise

Exercise demands a whole lot of energy in the form of glucose and carbohydrates, which are the simplest form of energy source. Therefore, it's important to fuel yourself up with your energy requirements. But it varies significantly from individual to individual.

The energy needs depend upon your gender, age, height, and weight, and also on the workout you're going to perform, and its intensity,

But you must consume a sufficient amount of carbohydrates, protein, and fat before beginning your exercise. Of all the three, carbohydrate is the most important, since it's processed more readily than fats and proteins.

As a generalized estimate from the American Orthopedic Society, an average athlete should consume 2-4 gram/kg of body weight of carbohydrates before the start. For endurance training and high-intensity workout that lasts for more than 2 hours, it is recommended to consume 7-10gram/kg of body weight/day. For protein, 1.2-1.7gram/kg of body weight/day is recommended, which means 20-30% of it should be consumed before the commencement of your workout. There are no set guidelines for fat, but 20-35% of calories should come from fat, with 10% coming from saturated fat.

So all in all, carbs are the main macronutrient you need to consume before your workout. Timing is important too, and you should eat at least 4 hours prior.

During The Exercise

During the exercise, it's important to maintain the energy level for sustained optimal performance. While short period exercises which last under an hour won't typically require you to consume anything except water, but when workouts last longer, focus on consuming at least 30 to 50 grams of carbs along with glucose water with added electrolytes. Hydrating every 15 minutes is a must.

After The Exercise

Post diet exercise should mainly focus on recovery and muscle building. After a moderate or an intensive workout, the cells of the involved muscles are at their best in processing glucose and carbohydrates. Therefore, within 15 to 30 minutes of workout, it is advised to consume 1.5 gram/kg of body weight. Also, consume 1-2 gram of protein which helps in repairing and building muscles. Drinking lots of water is crucial which aids in the recovery process.

Are Protein Shakes And Supplements Mandatory?

Many people who're into exercising, especially going to the gym, have a perception that protein shakes are mandatory for building muscles. However, that's not the case and varies based on your needs, type of exercise, and eating habits.

Protein is an important macronutrient which mainly helps in building muscles besides bones, skin, blood, and cartilage. It also supports the formation of many hormones and enzymes in the body. According to experts, daily intake of 0.8 grams of protein per kg of body weight per day is recommended.

For exercising people, it can go upwards to 0.9 or 1 gram. For professional athletes, it will be between 1.2 and 1.5. Most active individuals can easily fulfill their daily protein requirements by incorporating high-protein food into their diet. Foods like meat, fish, eggs, milk, cheese, soy, legumes, quinoa and are high in protein. Eating a sufficient amount of any of these can help you fulfill your daily protein requirement.

But protein powders are convenient to have, especially if you are constrained to meet their daily requirement because of any reason. It is easy to transport and easy to prepare. However, it is important to mention here that protein powder is different for men and women. Therefore, choose the one which meets your requirements perfectly.

While taking such protein supplements, it's important to measure the amount since an excess intake of it can pose long-term health risks like osteoporosis and kidney-related problems.

What Else Can I Drink Besides Water During The Session?

Water is sufficient for workouts lasting less than an hour. But if you're going to train for more than that (for close to 2 hours), and if the weather is humid with heavy sweating, then consider the following liquid intake:

- Sports drink

Sports drinks are high in glucose, electrolytes, and sodium -- the last two of which you lose mostly by sweating. Glucose is used by the cells, and a sports drink can help you refuel them. It is mandatory for endurance runners and sports that last longer like tennis, soccer, cricket, etc. But it is only recommended if you experience heavy sweating and your exercise lasts for close to 2 hours.

- Skimmed milk

Even though milk is discouraged to have during exercising, skimmed milk is recommended. Skimmed or semi-skilled milk have almost no fat in them, thus it doesn't upset your stomach. Milk contains essential minerals and vitamins. Thus, milk can help you in replenishing all the nutrients which you've lost during sweating. Not to forget it is high in protein and carbohydrates.

- Energy drink

Often mistaken for being the same as sports drinks, energy drinks are different in that they contain high levels of caffeine along with sugar. As the name suggests, they are just meant to boost energy but don't provide the electrolytes and sodium as sports drinks. As they cause a myriad of health-related problems, they're not usually recommended to replace sports drinks.

How Effective Are Marketed Vitamin And Mineral Supplements?

Just like protein powders, vitamins and minerals supplements are an absolute necessity. But you can easily hit your daily requirements by your diet. By consuming a variety of fruits and vegetables, nuts, cereals, you can easily fulfill your requirements. Furthermore, there is little evidence to suggest that they actually improve athletic performance or even aid in maintaining proper health.

Such supplements are only recommended when you have a deficiency of something, like Vitamin C, Vitamin A, potassium, etc. If you're not getting enough sunlight, then Vitamin D supplement is prescribed. Intake of any such kind of supplements should be consulted first by a dietician or GP.

Taking Care of Nutrition during Menopause: 5 Tips Plus 1

Menopause is an important phase in your life. Although it is nothing to be scared of, your body becomes prone to developing certain situations and diseases which can easily be handled with the help of a proper diet.

Here is how you can take care of your nutrition while on menopause while also avoiding weight gain:

- Consume enough calcium

Calcium is important, but it becomes all the more important when you approach menopause. This is why it is highly recommended to consume two to four servings of foods rich in calcium every day. You must consume fish, dairy products, broccoli, and legumes to ensure that you consume a minimum of 1,200 mg per day.

- Fruits and vegetables

Irrespective of your age, including enough fruits and vegetables in your diet is a must. It is highly recommended to have at least 4 cups of fruits and vegetables every day.

- Iron

Deficiency of iron and women go hand in hand. Thus, make sure that you consume enough iron every day. You can find iron in foods like nuts, fish, red meat, eggs, green leafy vegetables, and others. Aim to consume at least 8 milligrams per day.

- Drink water

We already stressed the importance of having enough water every day. According to the general rule of thumb, consume around 8 glasses of water every day to meet your daily requirements.

- Consume enough fiber

Consuming dietary fiber is important for our digestive health. Consume foods rich in fiber like fresh fruits and vegetables, cereals, pasta, bread, rice and so on to meet your daily requirement of 21 grams of fiber a day.

- Be physically active

It is highly recommended to stay physically active. You must, at least, perform the moderate-intensity exercise for 30 minutes on most days of the week. You don't have to hit the gym to exercise but simple physical activities like dancing, walking or gardening can do the trick.

Additionally, try strength-building exercises twice a week. This will not only help you in gaining rid of muscle mass, but it will also slowdown the process of losing minerals which will help you in fighting against osteoporosis.

Weight Gain with Menopause

More often than not, women end up gaining weight with menopause. This is all because of the lowering hormone levels. Women tend to lose muscles and gain fat, particularly in the belly area. If you are experiencing the same symptoms too, it is the right time to become more active and eat lesser calories.

Weight gain not only interferes with your body shape but it also leads to a range of health issues including high blood pressure, high cholesterol. Some women also develop insulin resistance which might lead to diabetes if not controlled properly.

To avoid this metabolic crisis, it is necessary that you make some changes in your lifestyle. Unfortunately, there are no quick fixes which will help you in reversing the change, but you can do your little bit, one step at a time.

Step2: Making Way for a Healthier Lifestyle

Now that you know leading a healthier lifestyle is important, you can't wait to live it. Yes? But how do you start? How do you start living healthily? Well, this is what I am going to talk about in this section.

I remember a few years ago I met an old woman. I frequently used to visit a café where she used to sell some magazines. On noticing that I am the regular visitor of the café, she asked me what do I like the most about that particular café. Without blinking an eye – I said coffee! And she replied with equal excitement that consuming so much caffeine is not just unhealthy, but expensive too. Defending my habit, I told her that it is a habit difficult to get rid of. To which she replied – "We first make our habits, and then our habits make us."

So true!

Healthy Habits Lead to a Healthy You

So you finally decided to make the transition? Are you all set to develop new healthy habits? To help you in this task of yours, here are a few habits that you must aim to inculcate. Rest assured, I will support you throughout the process by explaining how you can do it. I will talk about that in the next section.

For now, let's focus on various healthy habits that you must have:

- Start your day fresh

With fresh, I don't only mean taking a shower and getting ready but also making way for fresh beginnings. Had an unresolved fight with your spouse/mom/landlord yesterday? Or has an awful day at work?

No matter how bad your previous day was, today is a new day and start it afresh. Let bygones be bygones, and start your day on a positive note.

- Drink something warm in the morning

It is important to start your day with a fresh warm drink. It expels all the toxins out from your body, and also spreads positivity. How about having a glass of lukewarm water with lemon? In addition to cleansing your digestive system, this simple habit of yours will also boost your immune system and make your skin glow!

- Count to 10 before reacting

Pissed off? WAIT. Do not react. Count to 10, and you will be surprised to know that 10 seconds could be more than enough in gaining the required perspective. It helps you in getting rid of anger, and also provides you with rational arguments to put your point across.

- Put down your cell phone

Keep your phone consumption in check, and ensure that you only use it at the times of need. Using cell phones right before going to bed is a complete no. It interferes with your sleep cycle and distracts your time.

So keep your Facebook and Instagram scrolling for the next day.

- Avoid overdoing the booze

A few cocktails every now and then are fine, but overdoing it almost regularly is a strict NO! It can interfere with your personal life and can also lead to insomnia and weight gain. If certain reports are to be believed, it can also keep you at an increased risk of breast cancer.

- Don't skip your yearly gynecological appointments

Rest all can wait but do not ever give up on your yearly gynecological appointments. You might be busy, but it is actually important to take out the time and talk with your doctor regarding what is happening with your body.

- Quit smoking

I understand quitting smoking is not easier. It needs a lot of dedication, but believe me, in the end, it is worth all the efforts. If you become adamant enough towards your goal, you can quit smoking. It's harder in the beginning but once you stick to your goal for the first two days, the rest of the task will become easy.

- Reduce stress factors

When things that need to be done keep revolving around your head the whole day, it results in stress. Increased stress in your life makes you prone to various diseases like high blood pressure and heart strokes. Make sure you don't overburden your day with work. Further, exercise daily to eliminate stress and you will be happier.

- Walk whenever you can

This is the simplest healthy habit to inculcate. However, you would be shocked to know that the minimum number of steps that we all are required to walk daily is 10,000. Yes, you read that right. That seems impossible to achieve but we can get closer to it every day by walking whenever we can.

Stroll around as much as you can. You can keep a count on your daily steps by downloading step counter app in your mobile.

- Take the stairs

Choose to ascend or descend through the stairs instead of lifts and escalators. Introducing such small changes in life will keep you healthy. What's more, you will actually feel happy about accomplishing something that is for the wellbeing of your body. Essentially, you will also burn some extra calories, thus losing weight.

- Straighten your posture

What is the right posture? It is when your hips and back are in a straight line, your shoulders are lifted and your chest is out. We lose our right posture and swoop down low without even realizing. A right posture also brightness your personality and reduce the chances of back pain in the long run.

- Focus on your breathing for some time

Devote a small amount of time to focus on your breathing through meditating, doing yoga or just while sitting idle. Not breathing mindlessly but focusing on taking deep breaths actually provides good health benefits -- it lowers your blood pressure, heart rate, provides tranquility to your mind and reduces stress.

So take deep breaths whenever you are free next time.

- Get some sleep

The ideal amount of sleep time is 7 to 8 hours in the night. If you sleep lesser than this, you need to modify to your schedule. Proper timely sleep is important to start your next day afresh. It also helps in keeping your mood high, sharp memory and longevity of life.

- Tell someone about your health and fitness goals

It's not about flaunting but telling someone your health and fitness goals makes you more committed to achieving them and also motivates others. Inspire others in living a healthy life by communicating your health and fitness goals to others will make everyone lead a happy life.

So be the source of inspiration to others to lead a healthy life starting from now.

And the last but not the least, lose weight if you are overweight.

Now that you have a list of healthy habits in your hand, let's see how you can inculcate these habits into your lifestyle without breaking a sweat.

14 Easy Ways to Develop Healthy Habits

Undoubtedly, old habits die hard. You might already know that skipping breakfast is not good for health. But amid all the chaos, willingly or unknowingly, you often end up skipping the breakfast.

Sounds relatable? You are not alone! This is true for most of us.

Changing our habits is difficult, but there is nothing that you can't do. All you need to do is love the change. Bring the changes that you need in your life right now, don't wait to hit the rock bottom to wake up.

Here are 14tipswhich will help you in changing unhealthy habits, eventually if not immediately but definitely:

- Tip1: Identify your bad habits

Needless to say, you cannot bring about a change until and unless you identify the root cause of the problem. The best way to identify your bad habits is by enhancing your awareness. Keep a close eye on everything you do, the way you think, and the things you eat. You will surely start distinguishing the good from the bad.

While waking up early is good, skipping breakfast is bad. Staying productive throughout the day is good, but stressing yourself is bad. Taking care of yourself is good but biting nails unknowingly is bad. Bring your unconscious behavior to your awareness and identify all the problematic areas.

This doesn't mean that you need to feel guilty every other hour. We all have bad habits, and you are just taking the right step in ruling them out of your life. Don't forget to pat your back whenever you come across a healthy habit of yours!

- Tip2: Answer the 'Why'

You cannot motivate yourself to reach somewhere if you do not even know why you wish to go there in the first place. The same happens when you are trying to change your lifestyle. If your heart and mind do not know why they need the change, they will not stay with you for long.

Clear your mind and tell your heart why you have to make the switch. It can be that you wish to raise your self-esteem and confidence or you want to set an example for your kids. Whatever the reason, if you do not have the answer to your 'why', you are likely to lose your motivation.

- Tip3: Look at what you are getting out of it

As it turns out, every bad habit that we have tends to comfort us in one way or the other. The nails that you bite might help you in getting rid of the stress. The breakfast that you skip might help you in reaching the office 20 minutes earlier.

You will soon find out that all your bad habits are providing you with some sort of comfort in return. All you need to do is replace your bad habits with healthier outcomes.

- Tip4: Listen to your inner voice

So you are damn tired after teaching your kids, and attending an hour-long conference call? So you just stay up way too late to binge watch your favorite series on Netflix. You know you will be all exhausted and unproductive the next day, but somehow you feel attracted to this toxic schedule.

Your inner voice might signal you that this is not correct. This is when you have to respect your wisdom and listen to it, no matter what.

- Tip5: Replace your unhealthy habit with a healthy substitute

The best way to get rid of an unhealthy habit is to replace it with its healthy counterpart. What can you do instead of biting nails when you are stressed? Have a plan B ready for you. Next time, when you feel stressed and bite nails, simply inhale and exhale to the count of 10. Or maybe talk with your friends and family whoever comforts you the most.

Every time you make such healthy changes, acknowledge your efforts and feel proud. You can say to yourself "I just made a healthier choice, and I will keep making more such choices." Such simple acts of yours will replace bad habits with the healthy ones and all of this will flow subconsciously, without you forcing yourself to make the change.

- Tip6: Remove triggers

If keeping mayonnaise cheese in your refrigerator makes you crave for a pizza, stop storing cheese at home. If a certain friend of yours makes you drink, stop seeing them, at least for a while until you feel secure in your new schedule and habit.

It is essential that you pay closer attention to your environment and find out what triggers you, and what does not.

- Tip7: Visualize the changed you

Think about the changed you, the one who only has healthier habits. The one who wakes up early. The one who eats only the healthy stuff. And so on. Envision yourself with the new habits.

You might not see this coming, but this kind of visualization really works wonders. It creates positive vibes and spreads happiness. Other than that, it also wires your brain accordingly and helps you in moving ahead on the healthier track.

- Tip8: Keep your negative self-talk in check

All your negative thoughts have an adverse effect on your health. Thus, whenever you curse yourself or under-estimate yourself saying: "No one likes me", "I am fat" or "I am good for nothing" – monitor yourself.

Replace it with all the good and positive thoughts like I feel more confident, I am becoming healthy, and so on. Rewire and retrain your brain, and feel the difference, from day 1.

- Tip9: The colors of the company

You may not realize it, but you learn and adopt a lot from the type of people you live with. Your friends have a lot of influence on your life and habits. Thus, whichever practice you are trying to bring into your life, make some friends who are either on the same track or have already inculcated it in their lives.

It becomes easier to do something when you have a partner with you. That friend would be the biggest source of motivation for you when you feel like giving up or cheating. Surround yourself with people who share the same goals as you, or at least who do not make you deviate from your aim.

- Tip10: Do the to-do

Do you know that feeling where you put a tick mark besides an item on your checklist? How great and accomplishing that feels! It is a very happy moment when you tell yourself that you achieved something that you decided.

Follow this principle and apply it when you are developing a new healthy habit. Take a calendar and write down the things that you need to do in order to make that habit a part of your lifestyle. It would make you work harder to put a check-mark every day in the calendar.

- Tip11: One at a Time

Have you ever played Jenga? You can manage to win if you pull out the sticks one by one. But if you pull two or three in one attempt, the whole puzzle comes crashing down. That is the exact policy you should follow when you have a list of changes to make in your life.

Always focus on one habit at a time. Good health is achieved slowly. It would be harder for you to work upon three or four alterations in your lifestyle. You would not want to disrupt your normal life in order to bring in a new one. Changes come slow and take time.

It is not impossible or tedious to adapt to a new healthy lifestyle. If you are serious enough to bring some necessary and hygienic changes in your life, then these steps can be a great guide for you to move forward.

- Tip12: Keep it slow, but moving

Finding it tough to keep up with your newly developed healthy habits? Take baby steps, do not rush, but make sure that you maintain the momentum. You might have blocked out an hour to read a book but you need to attend your kid's school urgently. Make sure that you reschedule your habit to another time slot without giving up on it.

This will help you in reinforcing your new habit and wiring your brain accordingly. Make sure that you do not skip your habit even for a day or two. Once you do that, you will lose your momentum and you will be back to square 1.

- Tip13: Understand that it will take time

Developing new habits is not a child's play. You are going to fail drastically. Accept it. Rome was not built in a day. It might take several weeks for you to reflect on your habits, and follow them effortlessly.

- Tip14: Start small, achieve big

Do not try to achieve it all at once. You cannot suddenly accommodate a new habit into your settled life. Take your gym workout, for example. You cannot start with push-ups and planks. The initial weeks are for cardio and squats. You should start small and slow, and then pick up the pace.

Similarly, choose a healthy habit that is realistic and achievable. But again, start from the basics. For instance, assume that you chose to start going for a run every morning. Though you might be able to just walk or jog for a few days, in the beginning, you will find yourself sprinting after a month. Also, do not set your aims too high. It is not a smart decision to set aside two hours for a workout when you hardly find time to eat.

Step 3: How Our Body Reacts To Training, And More

Have you ever wondered why the same set of exercises is highly effective on your friend and not on you?

This is a common query we all have, especially when we gym with our friends.

One such query was put forward by my gym friend. She asked the instructor as to why pec decks don't work for her but they work immensely great for her friend. The instructor replied in a simple sentence – it is because of your body type.

So what does he meant by that? Let me explain.

Know Your Body Type and Optimize Your Lifestyle

In order to get the best results from your nutrition regimen, it is necessary that you know your body type to get visible results faster.

Technically, somatotype (body type) is an attempt to categorize humans based on three fundamental elements which are derived from the germ layers of embryonic development. These body types are important as these can later help in deriving the mental and personality characteristics of an individual.

This whole concept was theorized and popularized by American psychologist William Herbert Sheldon. He attempted to make a relation between body structure and behavior after observing that certain individuals with similar body composition carried certain behavior. His initial work was termed as Constitutional psychology, but it is now a neglected theory.

Even though the original theory is disputed and discredited, relative work carried out by his research assistants Barbara Heath, Lindsay Carter, Rob Rempel are still used at an academic level.

According to William Sheldon, there are three types of Somatotype:

- Endomorph

- Mesomorph
- Ectomorph

Each individual can be rated between 1 and 7 depending based on their body shape and structure. A rating of 7-1-1means that the person is pure endomorph, 1-7-1 means that the person is pure mesomorph, and 1-1-7 means that the person is pure ectomorph. All of these concepts and theories are detailed in Sheldon's book "Atlas of Men" which came out in 1954.

Let's discuss these three somatotypes in detail.

Three Basic Somatotypes

- Endomorph

Individuals categorized under Endomorph possess large and rounded body shape with wider hips and shoulder. Thus, they look shorter in height, plump, and visceral. The fat stored in their body is readily noticeable which gives them a rounded look.

Endomorphs find it difficult to lose weight and make changes to their body structure. Diet plan and physical activity seem to have no effects on their body composition. But this type of body is excellent in terms of power and strength. The body types of rugby players, power lifters, and strength athletes can be considered as an endomorph.

People with this body type are described as outgoing, cheerful, pleased, happy, sociable, affectionate, tolerant, complacent, lazy, greedy, and ungenerous.

- Mesomorph

Mesomorphs are the intermediate types. People with this body type are not as rounded as endomorphs and not as skinny or tall as ectomorphs. They are considered lucky because they tend to possess a noticeable muscular structure without even trying.

Their physiology includes larger frames, wide back, and narrow hips. Athletes in sports like basketball, soccer, baseball are considered mesomorphs. Their muscular structure allows them to perform at the peak level in their respective sports.

Mesomorphs are described as athletic, extroverted, authoritative, dominant, energetic, direct, assertive and strong in nature. So, they can be thought of as an aggressive group of people.

- Ectomorph

People falling under this category are naturally lean, slender, and tall in height, less muscular, flat-chested, and fragile. Although they possess muscles, muscles are seldom visible because of their tall height. Therefore, they're often called "lanky."

Ectomorphs often struggle to gain weight and make changes to their body composition. Going to the gym and being on a muscle mass gain diet seem to have little to no effect on them. They're often categorized as endurance athletes.

Based on their physical structure, they tend to have psychological traits like soft, gentle, soft-loving, non-assertive, quiet, sensitive, restrained, concealing, quirky, inferior, and the likes. So as with their body composition, they tend to be on the weaker side of things.

William Sheldon, an American psychologist, suggested that based on the shape and corresponding size, every human body can be categorized into three categories.

- Ectomorph- People with a skinny, lean figure, having difficulty gaining muscles
- Endomorph- People with fat, rounded shape body, having difficulty losing fat
- Mesomorph - People with a natural well-built figure, with excellent body metabolism

What do Somatotypes Mean For You?

Undoubtedly, you probably fall under one of the three categories mentioned above. Intuitively, you might ask what this means for you. First of all, there are certain perks of being in a certain somatotype category.

For example, ectomorphs who are born with a skinny framework are better positioned to practice aerobic exercises like running. This is natural since their longer limbs will help them cover more distance with the same effort. The lower body fat percentage also helps them move swiftly without having to carry excess weight. Same goes for endomorphs who can become better power lifters, thanks to their bulky composition.

But this doesn't mean that you're shackled to a certain body type for the rest of your life. In fact, many reputed distance runners weren't skinny at the beginning of their career or most power lifters didn't have the bulk as they seem to have now. That leads us to our next section: can your somatotype be changed?

Can Somatotypes Be Changed?

Knowing the category you belong to, you may wish to bring some changes to it. The ectomorph might wish to gain some muscles and endomorphic might wish of slimming down a bit.

It is worth mentioning here that while genetics might predispose you to a certain body structure, your lifestyle definitely has its own role to play. By incorporating certain lifestyle changes, you can change your somatotype effortlessly.

For example, most NBA players are tall which categorize them as ectomorphs. They're also fragile and weak, which shouldn't allow them to participate in the sports. But because of extensive round-the-year full-body strength training that they undergo at academies, they are able to gain strength and make muscles while their height remains the same. So they shift from an ectomorph to a hybrid ectomorph-mesomorph somatotype. Thus, with training, and a few changes in your eating habits, you can too go to a hybrid state and achieve your goals.

But it's easier said than done. It's not a short-term undertaking, but rather a long-term commitment. When you start off with altering your body structure, your body will adapt to the changing conditions and make it even harder for you. But the key is staying committed to the lifestyle changes and practicing them religiously.

Being born with a particular somatotype isn't a guarantee that you'll maintain the same body structure in the long run. An athletic stud with mesomorph frame can accumulate fat if the eating habits are not kept in check.

With the above information, you can certainly get to a lifestyle that's more in line with your body composition. By testing what works and what doesn't work for you is the best way to bring changes to your predisposed body structure.

How to Train the Right Way as Per Your Body Somatotype

When you have a good understanding of what body shape you were genetically born with, it's easier to meet your fitness goals.

Training for Ectomorph

In the case of ectomorphs, they're able to process carbs more readily into energy. In fact, the metabolism is so fast that all carbs get burned off quickly, and there's nothing to be left to be stored as fats. Another reason is their fast-twitch fibers are underdeveloped. The trick to adding more muscles is to increase the number of cells which surround these fast-twitch muscle fibers. But that's where the problem lies since ectomorphs develop such cells at a slower, that too after a lot of efforts.

But that's not to say it's an impossible feat. To gain muscles and weight, ectomorphs must focus on compound exercises rather can cardio-only workouts. Compound exercises focus on multiple muscles in one session, are intense, and hence stimulate the release of growth hormones.

Bicycle crunch, abs crunch, German volume training, jumping jacks and other compound exercises along with a few cardio workouts work best for ectomorphs.

Training for Endomorph

Problems endomorphs face is because their body is programmed to store excess fat. In fact, in terms of managing your weight and fitness is the hardest for this category of people. Most of this inability to lose weight more readily is hereditary, which experts suggest accounts for nearly 70% of BMI or Body Mass Index. The rest depends on their lifestyle and eating habits.

So to really change your somatotype, you need to incorporate exercise into your lifestyle. For the best fat loss results, high-intensity interval-based aerobic exercises are best. They demand a lot of energy within a short period of time. Sprinting, box jumps, skipping, along with few compound exercises will really tax your body. You have to pair it with a good eating habit consisting of complex carbs, fibers, whole foods, vegetables, and lots of water.

The overall aim here is to reduce the calorie intake and force the body to use its own fat reserves.

Training for Mesomorph

Mesomorphs are considered to have the best body types. As opposed to ectomorphs, they can easily add new muscles. And unlike endomorphs, they don't store excess fat, thanks to fairly good metabolism.

Just one thing mesomorphs have to take care of is maintaining that optimal level. Exercising regularly and having a balanced diet will do more than good.

If you, being a mesomorph, decide to bulk up a bit, it'll be easier for you. Any form of exercise ranging from cardio-workouts to aerobic training will be good. But most importantly, you should focus on your diet. Mesomorphs often take the perks for granted and get into a high-calorie diet.

How Fat Burns Inside Your Body

Fat is one of the energy sources for the body by utilizing which it keeps itself running.

Where fat is stored?

First, let's get where fat is stored straight. If your answer is whatever you eat goes right in your belly, then that's incorrect. Fat is present at every part of your body and is evenly distributed as per your weight. There might be some areas where it's seemingly more, but that's because of genetics and heredity.

The fat storage process goes something like this: When you eat food, all essential macronutrients like carbohydrates, protein, and fat gets converted into calories. They are spent on performing everyday activities and during exercises. The excess amount, however, gets stored in fat cells, known as adipocytes. These can increase and decrease in size depending upon the calories that are being left behind. If more calories are present, then fat cells will become larger in size. If the stored fat reserves are used, then it causes weight loss.

How our body gets energy?

Just hitting the gym and performing a hundred pushups is not enough to lose fat. First you have to understand how your body uses calories and from where you get them exactly.

When we eat something, the major energy source for the body comes from carbohydrates, proteins, and fat.

Long vs. short period exercise

If you're exercising for a shorter period of time at high intensity, then you're using carbs as fuel as it breaks down easily when compared to fats.

Fat burns when you exercise for a longer period of time, slowly and steadily. As fat provides the maximum energy, the body will break it down to have access to energy.

There's a switch which occurs from carbs to fats since carb stored in the body is limited. After you exercise for a significant amount of time, fats will get used up as energy when the body runs out of carbohydrates.

But this theory remains disputed with researchers suggesting that short period exercises don't show considerable fat-burning activities. According to them, short-period high-intensity workouts are more impactful.

The fat burning process

The fat stored in your body breaks down undergoing a complex process known as metabolism which is responsible for conversion of fat molecules into ATP, the molecule responsible for transporting chemical energy within cells.

When our body runs out of both glucose and carbohydrates, it triggers a chemical process in our body, and by that chemical process, fat or triglycerides are broken down into glycerol. Kidney and liver then absorb glycerol and break it down further to release energy. The byproduct of this chemical process is water, carbon dioxide, and heat.

To turn your body into a fat burning machine, you'd have to spend more calories than you consume. So it's a mix or balance between eating right and exercising right. As a rule of thumb, the more you exercise, the more calories you burn, and the less calorie-dense food you eat, the fewer calories body gets and stores.

Discover How Muscles React to Training

When it comes to building muscle strength, intense workout is the last thing that you should be thinking about. Too much intensive workout can prove to be redundant and therefore will be not as efficient in the overall growth of muscles. Stressing your muscles with the required amount of resistance and providing them with a sufficient amount of rest will help you develop muscles in the right way possible.

During training, your muscles are forced to perform a lot of contractions and relaxations. This leads to the formation of Microtears or Microscopic Tears in the muscle fibers. These muscle tears are the exact reason why you feel fatigued after a workout. Without muscle tears, it is almost impossible to improve the size, strength and capacity of the muscle. This is the reason why compound exercises are recommended, as they stress upon multiple groups of muscles rather than a single group. Compound exercises make you fitter and stronger.

Muscle tearing is nothing but the creation of lactic acid inside the muscle cells, due to the formation of energy. The lactic acid build-up also develops soreness within the muscles. This can last around 24 to 72 hours. This process is also termed as Delayed Onset Muscle Soreness or DOMS. The pain that is inflicted in this case will be much different than an injury pain. You should still be able to perform daily routine tasks and activities, unlike inflicted injury pain.

Also, soreness or DOMS is the perfect way to ensure that your muscles are getting built. Over time, the muscles will gain endurance and therefore the workout will prove to be less painful and the recovery might be quicker than usual.

Importance of Rest after Training

It is highly recommended to consume essential nutrients after workout - which should be loaded with carbohydrates, proteins and fats. Rest is another aspect of muscle growth. With the help of the essential nutrients and sufficient rest, the muscle tears will be rebuilt and the muscles will grow stronger and healthier.

The recovery process is carried out in the muscle cell where old tissues are replaced by newer ones. However, new muscle tissues can only be created if you take the right amount of nutritional raw materials, especially good amounts of protein. Even though there is no such straightforward rule for muscle recovery and it can differ from person to person - sleeping eight hours a day and taking off from workouts around 1-2 days per week should be perfect. Or you can also alternate your workout days and rest days as well.

Besides resting, you can also perform numerous recovery workouts as well, including yoga and swimming, which will help your muscles to recover and help you continue your workout for the next day.

Weights Would Make You Look Muscly... And Other False Myths!

Women all around the world are getting more and more aware of the need to be fit, and lead a healthy life. Well, if you are a beginner and are passionate about having a toned body, and are confused with a few aspects related to weightlifting, I am here to bust all the prevalent myths.

Starting with a simple myth which is prevalent everywhere- "big weight means big muscles". Well, this is completely untrue. Weight lifting never makes you huge and bulky. The purpose it serves is different from what some misguided fitness professionals will tell you at times. It does the opposite to what you think, it will not only burn all the visceral body fat but tone your body as well. The perfect shape of the curves can also be achieved via weight lifting. If done right, weightlifting could provide you with an attractive and perfectly toned body that you might be longing for long.

Thus, as far as weightlifting among women is concerned, countless myths and false facts have hidden the real fact. This is the reason that women often end up doing just cardio routine and develop a fear of weight lifting as well.

Further, it is very crucial not to get caught up in false marketing hype and advertisement. What is important is to stay focused and keep your diet in check. Along with it, follow the weight lifting routine which your trainer tells and guides you to do. You will definitely get fruitful results in some time.

It is also important to note here that you should not rely on drugs. One can have body supplements as directed by your fitness trainer or doctor but refrain from taking any drugs. Drugs can do more bad than good. They may be a cause of severe hormonal imbalance in your body leading to various health issues. Thus, relying on natural ways to get a perfectly toned body is recommended rather than depending on shortcuts.

In here, I will talk about false myths related to weight lifting for women. Thus, if you are thinking of weightlifting to get an attractive, fit and toned body, keep reading!

- Lifting weights would make you look muscly

Well, this classic myth is staying with us since forever! And, it doesn't seem to be going anytime soon. Firstly, if you include a few minutes of lifting weight in your exercise regime then, it will burn the extra fat off your body. There have been numerous studies which have concluded that rigorous resistance exercises and training help women in building strength.

Weightlifting is also found to improve the composition of your body. It also helps to improve body metabolism, eventually helping you to gain a perfectly cut body.

The issue here lies in the lack of knowledge. Most women who start with weight lifting exercise or gyming are not fully aware of the training required to put on the muscle weight. There are a different set of exercises which should be performed in order to gain a muscly-body.

The second reason as to why weight lifting won't make you look muscly is that- the level of testosterone level is significantly low in a women's body as compared to the man's body. Testosterone hormone is needed to gain muscle weight. Thus, if the level of hormones needed to build muscles is comparatively low, then there is no risk and fear of becoming muscly, as far as a women's body is concerned.

Having said this, there will be some change in the muscle weight due to the exercise but remember that the muscle weight is needed to achieve a trimmer and a leaner body. So, practice in a controlled manner.

- Cardio burns far more calories than weightlifting

There is no doubt that cardio is one of the easy, breezy, and cliché exercise which helps you in staying fit and healthy. But, if you are willing to weightlift, it is recommended to go for heavy resistance training. This will help you in improving your performance and gaining aerobic output.

Including cardio in your daily exercise routine may actually prevent you from getting a toned and lean body. This is because endurance training doesn't help you to gain a proportional physique or build any kind of strength. It is only better for a daily workout to have a healthy body and heart.

- Women need to use different protein powder than what men use

All those brands which sell protein powder with a pink box and write "for women" are just doing it as a marketing strategy. This is because in reality there is no such thing as different protein powder for men or women.

Women and men both can consume the same protein powder. There is no need for special protein powder for that. Obviously, there aren't any "female-friendly" ingredients which are separately included in protein powder for women. It's all a myth. The ingredients of all the protein powders are almost the same, only the percentage of use might differ.

The only difference which is encountered as far as protein powder or body supplements are considered is- the dosage, which may vary for both men and women. It also depends on the fact, that what you want to accomplish while you are training. It can be either protein, carbohydrates, fat or calories. Thus, talk to your trainer. Find out what your body needs and then look for high-protein, low-carb or low-fat protein powder accordingly. Don't get carried away by high-end advertisements or market strategies. Be an informed and aware consumer.

- All you need is only lightweights

Well, when you start, not only women but even men should start with light weights and practice with them for a few initial days. This is recommended so that your body gets a chance to adjust to the change. It provides your body with a good understanding of how to manage resistance. When this is achieved, slowly start to increase the weights in a progressive manner, so as to get a lean body.

Don't get stuck with light weights, as it is recommended to challenge your body for better results. Some women just get stuck to light weights thinking, it will tone their body. But, get this straight that there is no such thing as toning. The entire process of getting a lean and trimmed body is a goal which can be achieved only with the right set of weightlifting exercises routine and recommended body supplements. Knowing your body is the key here.

- The more your age, the more dangerous it becomes to lift weights

Well, this is one of the most prevalent myth out there in the world. In fact, it is contrary to what people think or say. The fact is that older women need to exercise fundamentally, to stay fit and fine as they grow old. This is a known fact that as your body grows old, you are at a risk muscle and bone deterioration, reduction in body flexibility and all this lead to a slower metabolism. Now, at this stage and point of time if there is one thing which can help you immensely is a proper exercise routine. One very important thing to note here is that-weightlifting helps you to slow down the aging process and also, helps to keep your body in perfect shape.

Thus, it is recommended to include strength-based training and exercise as a part of your daily routine. Women who are approaching their menopause are more prone to have bone-related issues. In such a situation, exercises like weightlifting can help women in boosting the strength of their joints and tendons.

This can have a profound effect on your overall day to day life. A women's day to day life can be tiresome as they have to do a range of tasks. So, try to steal some time for yourself in such a busy life. This includes taking care of yourself, especially your body. Weight lifting also reduces the risk of injuries and falls which become frequent as you age.

Thus, if you are planning to start with weightlifting anytime soon, remember not to believe the above-mentioned myths and have proper facts and knowledge before you start with the training process. As a matter of fact, more women should get into weightlifting and make it a part of their lifestyle.

Exercising During Periods: What a Great Idea!

It's a myth! Yes, not exercising during periods as that can aggravate your menstrual cramps is disbelief. Doctors have opinionated that exercising when you are on your period can actually help you overcome your pain to an extent.

However, there are some dos and don'ts involved. There are certain exercises that must be performed during your periods. So, next time when you are on your period you have no excuses to avoid your daily workout.

Here is how you can do that.

1. Aerobic exercises or cardio

The key is to let your body release endorphins as they can help you in getting relief from cramps and headache. Thus, including light cardiovascular exercising is beneficial. It will enhance the blood flow in your body and provide you with relief from aches and pains.

Some of the cardiovascular exercises that you can easily perform at home include brisk walking, jumping squats, jump rope, planks and the like. However, it is highly recommended to workout only for a shorter period of time. Keep it lighter than you usually do in your normal days.

2. Strength training

Strength training refers to lifting weights. During periods your muscular power is increased. This provides you with an ability to lift weights easily. This is because estrogen levels are lowest during periods. However, don't lift heavier weights as this can trigger muscular cramps.

3. Stretching and balancing

Stretching can reduce your cramps and lengthen muscles. Performing simple stretching exercises like touching your hand to your feet without bending your knees proves to be beneficial during your menstrual cycle. Don't over strain by stretching more than what you are capable of at this time of your month.

4. Walking

Walking is another exercise that can be easily incorporated in your workout when you are on your periods. You can walk up to a speed that does not add discomfort to your body.

5. Swimming

Swimming is usually out of option during periods for all the obvious reasons. However, a relaxing dip in the pool can actually help you in relieving pain and eliminating fatigue. Adding swimming as a part of your daily workout session can diminish the pain you usually experience during your bloody days.

6. Deep breathing

The next exercise that can actually help you calm your nerves while you are on your period is deep breathing. Breathing deeply as part of your workout or during meditation enhances the blood circulation in the body. This, in turn, helps you in fetching quick relief from your period pain.

7. Sex

Having sex during your periods seems gross but you will really thank your partner after doing so. Orgasming releases a chemical called oxytocin which contracts the muscles of your uterus and this provides you relief from cramps. We all are aware of the benefits of orgasm. Not only it cures cramps but it is also beneficial in reducing mood swings, irritations, and period stress.

8. Dance

Dance it all out during your periods! If you are feeling pathetic lying in bed and holding your stomach all day long, it's time to get up and kick that period fatigue out of your system by dancing on the rhythms of your favorite song or by just watching out and following some Zumba videos. Dancing will lift your mood by eliminating stiffness from your body.

So these were some of the exercises that can be followed during the time of your periods.

These were the dos of exercising during periods. It's equally important to know the don'ts i.e. the exercises you should definitely strike off from your workout session during your periods and things to keep in mind while exercising.

- Studies show that there are increased chances of knee ligament injury, known as an ACL tear, during your menstrual cycle, so you should avoid excessive actions like jumping and skipping that can make you lose your body balance while landing.
- Don't perform inversion-type poses during your periods as that can put pressure on your uterus and can worsen your cramps.
- While doing any of the exercises, if the pain doesn't seem to improve but is getting worst, stop exercising immediately and rest.
- Also, if you are exercising during your periods, you have to take extra care of hygiene by changing your clothes and sanitary pad or whatever feminine

product you are using after you are done exercising.

Exercising During Pregnancy? With The Right Precautions...

Pregnancy brings a lot of changes to your body. Your tastes, likings, appetite, and strength are all altered. No woman's journey through the nine months is the same as others. Each one has her own set of issues and experiences. It is highly possible that what you were able to do comfortably before, might be painful and troublesome now that you have conceived.

Therefore, it is very important that you keep your doctor in the loop before bringing a change in your lifestyle during these months. Every discomfort, pain or irregularity that you notice must be confirmed with your gynecologist to ensure a healthy baby. And this specifically holds for exercising.

Your Body During Pregnancy

Whether you used to exercise before or not, it is a completely different thing to do it once you are pregnant. Every woman has a different body that may react differently to induced physical stress. Even before starting to lift those weights, consult your doctor to get the right advice. The needs and requirements of your body vary with each trimester. What might be benefiting you in the first one, may be harmful and uncomfortable during the second.

One most important thing that you must follow throughout the nine months is to keep your blood pressure below 140bpm. Going above this number can be dangerous for your baby.

- Exercise and First Trimester

Your first trimester is the time when you are tired all the time. You find it difficult to catch a break from the morning sickness, fatigue, and sore breasts. It is likely that your body itself would not allow you to attend the gym or any workout sessions. Your gynecologist might ask you to refrain from putting your body under any strain in the first three months of pregnancy.

If you had been training regularly before, then you might not want to stop. You can lift weights using slow and controlled movements. Avoid any jerks and sudden movements to your abdomen. Keep breathing throughout the workout and stop immediately if you start feeling unwell.

- Exercise and Second Trimester

You should prefer lifting weights while staying seated. It is also advised to refrain from standing for long periods. Once you are in the fifth month of your pregnancy, your baby bump will start to alter your center of gravity. This makes you tilt your back to maintain a comfortable posture while standing or exercising. DO NOT give in to the temptation.

Using your back for support after 16 weeks can press the vena cava. This major vein can limit the oxygen supply of your baby and make you feel dizzy or lightheaded.

Eventually, you will need to switch to even lighter weights and decrease the repetitions.

- Exercise and Third Trimester

Your bump will start getting in the middle of any equipment that you pick up. This makes you prone to knocking your bump accidentally with the weights. It would be, therefore, best for you to switch to free weights training and yoga. Avoid bending down to pick up weights. Do not lift weight either.

Area-Specific Exercises

You would know that there are exercises that focus on specific areas of your body. For example, doing crunches helps reduce belly fat and build abs. Here is a helpful list of exercises and the body parts that they affect after you have conceived.

- Upper Middle Back

Seated Cable Back, LatPulldown- Your breasts get bigger when you are pregnant, which makes your shoulder round forward. It is important to strengthen the shoulder muscles to counteract the slump.

- Chest

Seated Chest Press- Your upper body needs good muscle balance in pregnancy, and this can be done by working your pecs.

- Lower Body

Leg extension and seated leg curl- Your thighs and calves need to stay strong to bear the weight of your belly and support the pregnancy.

- Back

Planks- You are going to experience a lot of back pain as the baby makes its space inside you. Planks can be very helpful in preventing pregnancy-induced back pain.

The 'STOP' Symptoms

Your body always sends you signals when something is wrong. You need to be careful enough to identify and listen to them. You need to stop exercising immediately and consult your doctor the moment you experience any of the below symptoms:

- Bleeding from the vagina
- Dizziness
- Lightheadedness
- Chest pain
- Headache
- Out of breath
- Muscle weakness
- Swelling or pain in the calves
- Painful contractions in the uterus

- White fluid excretion

Precautions during Weight Training

- Lifting heavy weights is a big no for you. Switch to lower weights and do not resort to excessive workout. The idea is to maintain your blood pressure and heartbeat.
- Certain positions that make you exhale without any air must be avoided completely. This is necessary to ensure that your baby gets enough oxygen.
- Make sure that you tighten and squeeze the muscles of your pelvic floor before lifting a weight. A loose pelvic floor might hurt your bladder while you exercise.
- Try to keep away from doing exercises that can make you fall. Replace the unstable workout positions with those where you can maintain proper contact with the ground.
- Choose a cool and indoor workout place instead of going out in the heat. Your body already remains at a higher temperature during pregnancy. It is better to keep away from excessive heat conditions.

Alternatives to Weight-Training Exercises

A bit of physical exercise is always good for the body during nine months of pregnancy. While lifting weights may not be for everyone, there are many options for you to choose from to keep your body active. These are:

- Walking
- Swimming
- Yoga
- Pilates
- Aerobics
- Dance

Keeping your body physically active during pregnancy is an important and healthy thing to do. It eases your delivery and reduces the chances of a caesarian section. But everything needs to be done after keeping your doctor in the loop.

Exercising During Menopause? It's a Must!

Every woman is different and so is her experience with menopause. For some, it arrives early and for some it takes time. For some, it comes like a wrecking ball but for others, it might just be less dramatic.

Here is the good news. By making small changes in your life, you can actually change the way menopause is treating you. You choose not to talk about it with anyone but I can hear your plea.

By making a few lifestyle changes like exercising along with keeping control of your diet, menopause won't be that severe for you. Here are a few exercises which you can do during menopause to ease up the symptoms.

- Strength training

The most important and underperformed exercise at the age of menopause is actually strength training. During menopause, there is a loss in the level of estrogen in your body which interferes with your ability to hold down urine. Strength training provides the needed strength that can help in building the pelvic floor stronger. This way, it reduces the risk of urine incontinence.

Not only this, loss of estrogen makes your muscles weaker. This makes you prone to developing osteoporosis. Also, some women experience back pains and joint pain during their menopause. Strength training can help a lot in this regard.

It helps in making the bones and muscles stronger and improves your inner body strength. Women during menopause should avoid lifting heavy weights. A lightweight lifting session for three minutes five times a week will make a huge difference. Start the process by holding lightweights such as dumbbells. Increase your capability as your strength continues to build up. You can also choose to go for deadlifts, sleds, barbell and the like for the best results.

- Yoga

If strength training still feels out of the league for you, go for yoga and meditation. As mentioned before, the menopause symptoms are different for every woman, you will need to find remedies that work best according to your symptoms. The best exercise you can choose to make your body relax is either through deep breathing, meditation or yoga.

Certain poses of yoga can help you calm your nerves and provide you relief from the symptoms of menopause like hot flashes, fatigue and mood swings.

- Dancing

This is another way to fight against your menopause symptoms. If dancing makes you feel alive, it is highly recommended to dance your heart out instead of burning some carbs over a treadmill! Do whatever gets you moving and don't let your muscles die and lose flexibility.

- Make use of cardio machines

Cardio workouts are really helpful in relieving the menopause symptoms. If you are tired of running on the treadmill or bored of the same cardio exercises, you should not forget the cardio machines like StairMaster and

Elliptical. Any sort of running will be helpful in reducing the risk of cardiovascular disease. The estrogen which is responsible to protect you from any heart diseases drops down during menopause which increases the risk of CVD. Embracing cardio exercises in your lifestyle can eliminate such risk. It will also help you in living a healthier life.

- Zumba

Will you love to move your body on the eclectic beats of Latin songs along with everyone else in the gym? When you watch others do Zumba, you will definitely be enchanted by its energy and feel. It's age no bar and interesting way to get your body moving and keep it working perfectly.

- Vigorous housework

Managing your daily house chores such as dusting, gardening or DIYs can't be termed as vigorous housework. Doing housework does burn some calories but not to the extent of traditional exercises. Though housework involves more body movement depending on the way you choose to perform your duties, housework or yard work has to be really vigorous to a point that it palpitates your heart beat faster. That is when it will be beneficial.

Other than these, Menopause also results in loss of lean muscle mass. By following some special cardio exercises, you can maintain your lean muscle mass. Just muscle mass is not enough but it has to be strong and rigid.

Some of the activities to follow during menopause include:

- Lunge walking

Lunge walking can actually help you in maintaining the stability of your body. In here, you need to bend your knees in such a way that it forms a right angle and one of your leg's knee touches the ground. Practicing lunge walking is helpful in toning your muscles.

- Push-ups

Perform push-ups by involving your chest as much as possible. Make use of an elevated surface such as a box or wall to widen your movement.

- TRX rows

This is another interesting way to build up your muscles and keep them lean. It provides full body movement and an adjustable scale for pull-ups. It includes balancing your body weight by stretching ropes held up through your hand.

It is good for boosting your muscle strength and for keeping your back straight.

These were some of the exercises that can be done by a woman during their menopause and can eliminate their dreadful symptoms to an extent. Believe me, menopause symptoms can be tough, but you are TOUGHER! Stick to the right lifestyle, and perform the right set of exercises, and YOU CAN DO IT!

Step 4: Design your Own Workout Session and Become your Own Trainer

Workouts are essential, and so are gym trainers. They know how to tone your body and which exercises can get you back into shape. If you are trying to lose weight, they guide you towards the best mix of cardio and weight workout. But wouldn't it be more convenient and independent if you knew the right exercises yourself? It is like being well-acquainted with the gears and functioning of a car before you take the driver's seat yourself.

The day you enter a gym, you will be easily able to categorize the population into two- the cardio lovers and the weight lifters. In other words, you will find some people on the treadmill, bikes, elliptical machines, and others doing bench presses, lifting weights, and lifting more weights. A perfect workout is a combination of cardio and strength training sessions since each has its own benefits and functions.

In this section, I will tell you how you can design your own program. I don't recommend having a stringent plan because, more often than not, women hardly stick to it.I have never seen a normal client, not an athlete whose job is athletics but a normal client with a real life, who has managed to follow a program for more than 3 or 4 weeks.

Shit happens, sooner or later, people get sick, and their children get sick, there are anniversaries, weddings, graduation parties, where they indulge in eating.There are business trips and people take vacations, so they are forced to leave the gym for days or weeks...Or they can simply go through a period of stress, a family crisis or a period of poor physical fitness.

Therefore, the only rule that you should have is to set a realistic goal within three months and try to write down a rough schedule to reach that goal.It is important to acknowledge the fact that during the quarter there will be distractions, more or less serious reasons to deviate from the program. Consequently, the program will have to be corrected, not your life.

And the coach,whose job is to remove stress from your life, not to add more,is there to help.

So, ask himto help you plan your programming.

Cardio or Strength Training: Which is Better?

Cardio Training

Cardio is short for 'cardiovascular' which means relating to the heart and blood vessels, which is exactly what cardio training aims at. When you are doing a cardio exercise, your capillaries deliver more oxygen to cells in the muscles, therefore burning more fat than usual. It is good to feel your heartbeat rising up because that is when your heart is becoming stronger. You should push yourself to complete a lap even when you are out of breath.

Some of the most effective cardio training workouts are-

- Walking
- Elliptical
- Running
- Cycling
- Riding a Bike
- High Intensity Interval Training (HIIT)
- Climbing and Descending Stairs
- Jumping Rope
- Rowing
- Swimming
- Circuit Training

HIIT involves doing a high-intensity workout for a short period of time and then resting for that same period. A continuous pattern of such intense training can burn a huge amount of fat and calories. The right amount of cardio training should be at least 150 minutes per week at the minimum. The maximum depends on your body and endurance. Another tip is not to use the treadmill just for walking or running, but rather jogging and running at an incline to get the most benefits out of it.

Yays& Nays

A cardio training session has many benefits for your body.

- The exercises and intense sessions burn the fats and calories at fast rates, thus helping you to lose weight.
- Since it works more efficiently than before, you get a stronger heart.
- The increased blood flow and efficient delivery of oxygen to the muscles lowers the blood pressure and cholesterol levels in the body.
- Putting your body under intense stress releases endorphins that reduce stress and depression.
- A stronger heart reduces the risk for a stroke or any other heart disease to a great level.

But the positives come with some drawbacks.

- If your workout just includes cardio training, your body goes into a calorie-deficit state. This makes you lose muscle mass since your muscles become the fuel for the body in that state.
- Your body and mind both get exhausted from intense cardio sessions. This increases the risk of fatigue and injuries.
- After some time, your body adapts to your regular routine of cardio workouts and stops responding to it. In this case, it becomes harmful for you since your body starts storing fat instead of burning it.

Strength Training

Unlike cardio, strength training is about going against the reflexes and using muscular force against resistance. It involves making the muscles work against an external resistance to increase their strength, tone, mass, and endurance.

Over time, your body muscles adapt to this resistance and become more elastic and flexible. You can use free weights (dumbbells, barbells, hand-weights), weight machines, resistance bands, or even your own body weight (push-ups, squats, planks, sit-ups) to build your muscles and get stronger by adapting to weight lifting exercises.

Most weight lovers begin their workout sessions with squats, sit-ups, and push-ups and then move forward with the weight training. Also, strength training should not be confused with powerlifting or bodybuilding. While strength training boosts your general strength, power lifting or bodybuilding is generally pursued by athletes to optimize their performance.

It is always recommended not to work the major muscle groups (abdominal muscles, back, buttocks) on back-to-back days. One area a day with some supervision is the best way to work out with the weights, and this is how we have designed our program. Since the muscles are exposed to lack of air and intense workout during weight training, it is good to drink plenty of fluids for better performance and recovery. The workout should be progressive in nature so that the muscles can adapt to the new routine and maximize the benefits.

Yays& Nays

The good consequences of strength training are-

- The contracting of muscles against a resisting force makes them stronger and toned.
- Aging leads to loss of lean muscle mass and many other issues in bones and joints. Strength training preserves or increases muscle mass, strength, and power that are helpful for the health of bone, joint, and muscles in the long run.

- Just 30 minutes of weight training gives more strength to postmenopausal women with low bone mass.
- A strength training session improves your balance, posture, and coordination of the body. It also strengthens your immune system, thus keeping you from catching chronic diseases.

There is also another side of the coin.

- Some weight lifting exercises can have anaerobic moments which are not healthy for some hearts.
- Weak muscles are very prone to minor fractures in the back, therefore it becomes a necessity to make the journey as progressive as possible.
- You could suffer from muscle pain if you lift weights and expose your body to intense resistance.

The Right Mix is the Best

Strength and cardio training both have their own good and bad sides. Though the individual dark sides cannot be overlooked, you can easily combine the yays of both pieces of training to get the maximum benefits.

You can approach the combination in two ways.

1. Your first choice is to take up the two workout sessions on alternate days. That means cardio training on

Mondays, Wednesdays, and Fridays, and strength training on Tuesdays, Thursdays, and Saturdays. If you work out on Sundays too, you can dedicate it to yoga or for the recovery of your muscles.

2. The other option is, to begin with, cardio and end with weight lifting. You have fresh legs when you enter your gym which makes it easier for you to make the most out of a cardio session. Intake of fluids recharges and prepares your body and you can then begin lifting weights and have an intense session. In my view, this is the best option that you should choose to go with. This will help you in enjoying the advantages of both sessions.

But whichever way you opt to go, listen to your body for any signals that suggest stopping. Do not continue when there is a clear sign that something is going wrong. Talk to your trainer or a doctor, if need be.

Aerobic & Anaerobic Exercises

Science classes at school would have taught you that aerobic and anaerobic are related to the presence and absence of oxygen respectively. Thus, the exercises related to these states are related to oxygen levels in the body. You feel full of energy and out of it while working out. Some light workouts keep you relaxed, whereas intensive ones take your breath away.

Aerobic exercises need energy, and this is obtained from glycogen and fat stored in the body. Aerobics causes low levels of exertion in the body which does not produce lactic acid (responsible for fatigue). The benefits of these exercises are similar to cardio training, since it mostly involves swimming, biking, and running.

Anaerobic exercises make you run out of breath and you find yourself struggling to get a hold of your breath. Your body produces lactic acid in the body which raises the level of fatigue and discomfort. This is why these intense workout sessions should take place in short intervals. Strength training is the best way to get the most benefits of anaerobic exercises.

It can be seen that cardio training is aligned towards aerobic exercises while strength training is towards anaerobic. The human body needs a little of both to have strong muscles, right body shape and posture, strong immune system, and a healthy heart. This is why it is advisable to include both pieces of training in your workout sessions.

First Time at the Gym? Some Tips and Slangs...

The mirror will tell you when it is time to finally join a gym. There would be signs like side tires, weight gain, distorted curves, unwanted fat and loss of stamina. You will finally be able to convince yourself that it is very important to stay in good shape and health. If you have come to the realization and are eager to embark upon your fitness journey, then there are some things you should know beforehand.

There are some terms and information that every beginner should be familiar with on the first workout day. It is like knowing the theory part before you enter into a practical laboratory to perform experiments. You will not feel like an amateur or confused about what is going around if you know the basic pre-requisites.

When you begin on the first day, your trainer will ask you to do an exercise for a number of reps and sets. It is, therefore, important for you to know what these terms mean.

The Term "Reps"

The word reps is short for repetitions- the number of times you repeat an exercise. For example, when the trainer asks you to perform 15 reps of pushups, you are supposed to do 15 pushups. If you perform 20 squats, then you have completed 20 reps of squats. It is just the count of each time you move your body.

In the beginning, the number of reps for each exercise remains low, since your body muscles need to adapt to the exertion. Once your body stops hurting from intense workouts, the reps count will go up. Your trainer will know how many reps to allot you for each exercise, and when to change the number. They are experts in knowing the time taken for a woman's body to adapt to the physical exertion.

Females have constraints like menstrual cycles, pregnancy, weak back support, etc. This means that trainers cannot be careless about the amount of physical exertion they put you through. You have to perform just the right number of reps so that you do not end up harming your bodily function. Your workout has to be dedicated to strengthening muscles, losing fat and toning the body. It is best to listen to your trainer and not exceed the number of reps just because you have the energy to.

The Term "Sets"

A set is a collection of repetitions or reps of an exercise that you do in one stretch. For example, when your trainer asks you to do 3 sets of15 reps of squats, you are supposed to perform 15 squats, rest for a minute or two, do another 15 reps, rest, and finish with the last 15 repetitions. The common language in a gym is 'do 3 sets of 15', that means the word reps is skipped and is assumed to be present.

Trainers usually ask you to do alternate sets of two or three exercises that focus on two different body parts, so that the muscles get enough time to recover. The alternate set approach allows you to work out more and achieve maximum results. In this, you perform given reps of one exercise and follow it up with a set of a second exercise. This process goes on until you have completed the asked number of sets of both the exercises. Recovered muscles allow you to work out in a better way and with more energy.

Importance of Sets & Reps

This concept of sets and reps is important for an organized and structured workout session. When you know that 15 reps of a certain exercise need to be done, you push yourself towards that number. When you are not counting and just performing the exercise, you stop the minute you feel exertion or pain. It is essential to have a goal to push yourself towards the ultimate aim. Unless you have something to aim at, you would not be able to find the motivation to go on.

Think about this, in a set of 20 reps of pushups, if you get tired on the 16th pushup, what makes you go on? The fact that you only have to push your muscles to 4 more pushups gives you the motivation and energy to complete the set. This is why it is important to set a goal in the form of sets and reps for each exercise. An organized workout always gives the maximum results.

Tips to Optimize a Workout Session

If you are working out for building muscles, it is best to use slightly heavier weights instead of lighter ones. You can keep the repetitions as low as 3 sets of 8 reps, but the weights used in the exercise should not be very light. They should be heavy enough to make you struggle to complete the last rep, but not that heavy that you face physical problems. Your trainer would be able to recognize your endurance levels and will guide you about which weights would best suit your body needs and strength.

In contrast, if your workout is focused on muscle toning, you should either use light weights or no weights. All the exercises focused on toning should be done in 3 sets of 12-15 reps each. The resting time between each set should be limited to just 60 seconds and not more. Over time, when you are aiming at increasing the strength and endurance of your muscles, the resting time between sets should be set at 30 seconds at the maximum.

When you are a beginner, it is important that you stick to the instructions of your trainer and not push your body towards excessive exertion. It takes time for your body muscles and functions to adapt to physical stress. Complete the number of sets and reps as the trainer asks you, and avoid putting your body under intensive stress. Give it time to get accustomed to the physical exercise.

Not-to-do List

Before you even step into the gym, you must know what you are there for. You know your body the best, and only you can realize which areas need to be toned and where you need to lose fat from. Do not be clueless about your workout needs.

Never eat and exercise. If you just had food, take some time to digest it, and then proceed to the gym. Exercising on a full belly causes ingestion. Your body needs at least 2 hours after you have food to get ready for physical exercise. When you exercise with an empty stomach, you burn the maximum amount of fat.

Do what your trainer asks you to. Do not get intimidated or impressed while watching other people work out. They can be at advanced levels of training and their goals might be different. Just focus on yourself and your body. Ask your trainer what is best for you, and do not hesitate in asking for help when you cannot complete a set.

Sum-Up

Workout sessions can be really fun if you do it correctly and with enough motivation. Sets and reps are designed for your convenience and help. Take your work out seriously, and you get a shape that all friends would envy.

Equipment, Machines and Accessories: How to Use Those Strange Objects without an Engineering Degree!

Weight loss regimen is not complete unless it is accompanied by an intense workout plan. You can lose all the weight you want; but in the absence of proper exercise, you won't come out of it looking any good.

This is why I am here with all the details regarding the best equipment that you can use to aid your weight loss, along with details about how they're used.

Dumbbells

Dumbbells allow you to exercise each limb individually, a feature that is extremely helpful for improving your strength available in your less-dominant side. A few exercises also make use of stabilizer muscles, since every dumbbell workout does not have to have a fixed path. With the right exercises, dumbbells are also useful for working out your core muscles.

Pros

- Dumbbells are highly portable and can be stored at any location without a hitch. Regardless of whether you're at the beach, at home or simply just hankering for a quick workout session, you can always store a pair of dumbbells in your car or your home. They are highly portable and can be used in almost any place without a problem.

- They can be used in many ways for engaging and augmenting chest pecs, biceps, triceps and other muscle systems. There are a number of exercises out there that can be used for strengthening various core muscles throughout your body. Pecs, biceps, triceps, every muscle can be augmented using dumbbells.

Cons

- Dumbbells tend to lose their effectiveness as you advance through training, proving to be not-so-efficient as you get better. Once you've been exercising regularly, your abilities get better until you no longer find the same dumbbell to be challenging. That means, having to upgrade to more expensive and heavier dumbbells, which can be a waste of money.
- Upper limit dumbbells may not be challenging enough due to the lack of heavier options. Most dumbbells peak out at around 90 pounds, after which you will have to resort to gym

equipment. While dumbbells are good for the casual gym goer, it is unlikely to be of much use once you've crossed a certain physical strength barrier.

Barbells

Barbells are classified under free weights and consist of a metal tube, usually 5-7 feet in diameter, with removable weights on each end which can be added or removed, as per user choice. There are many types of barbells, including:

- Olympic Barbells
- Standard Barbells
- Cambered Barbells
- Fixed Barbells

Barbells come equipped with clamps or collars that ensure user safety. These can prevent accidents by preventing plates from slipping in case you lose control and tip the bar in one side. A leading cause of gym accidents is due to people not using the collar safely enough.

Pros

- Better weightlifting is possible compared to dumbbells. While dumbbells have maximum limits and can strain you out faster, using barbells can help you lift relatively heavier weights.
- Stabilizer muscles get actively engaged. These muscles are vital for aiding

proper movement. They ensure that you can hold huge amounts of weight without losing your stability.

- Several muscle groups are engaged at once. Shoulders, triceps, chest pecs are just some of the muscles that are engaged as you work out using barbells.

Cons

- Range of motion is restricted
- Certain muscles may not be trained well

Kettlebells

Kettlebells are the next big step after you're done with barbells and dumbbells. While the latter may be good for basic, the former lets you implement several new dynamic workout moves.

Kettlebells have a teardrop design with a large handle that can encourage jerks, swings, and presses. These are highly efficient fitness tools and may aid core-intensive and incredibly potent full body workouts.

Workouts involving kettlebells may include sumo squats, clean & press, and swings. Using kettlebells can help you with your cardio, endurance, power and strength workouts, thereby improving your fitness in all aspects.

However, not everyone can learn to use kettlebells effectively on their first. It is recommended that you engage a trainer to guide you through the initial stages.

Pick a kettlebell that has a solid casting and secure grip for optimal performance.

Pros

- These are an effective form of free weights that can provide effective resistance. They can enable massive fat loss in no time.
- Hamstrings and lower back muscles can be engaged effectively.
- Kettlebells, like dumbbells, are highly portable and can be used in any location without requiring much setup.

Cons

- While engaging lower back and hamstring muscles, care must be taken to execute the exercise well. Otherwise, you might end up with injuries.
- Once you've turned stronger, kettlebells may not provide ample benefits.
- Unless used properly, with the right techniques, you're better off sticking to dumbbells at times.

Seated Leg Press

These machines are useful for those looking to master movements before working out with heavy-duty barbells. They allow users to get a lay of the land and warm up their leg muscles.

There are often 2 seated leg press machines to pick from.

In one, you have to rest against horizontal plates by sitting straight and bending your legs. This machine is operated by straightening the legs, which pushes the body away up from these plates. You get to choose the weights you go against by sticking one pin into the weight stack.

With the other machine, you get to sit at angles which put your feet towards a platform that's above the head. This machine is operated by you pushing away via straightening of your legs. Resistance is increased by using weight plates which are loaded onto the machine.

Pros

- Useful for those recovering from an injury or for beginners.
- Useful for working out specific muscles like glutes, quads or hamstrings.
- Weights can be quickly adjusted while lifting.
- Safety is ensured along with optimal muscle augmentation.
- Recommended for fat-loss exercises.

Cons

- Can cause the body to have a propensity for injuries.
- Supporting muscles in ankles, hips, and knees are not fully engaged.
- Not very useful for muscle stability and all-round body development.

LatPulldown

When done right, this exercise can present formidable benefits. However, most people fail in implementing the right technique. For effectively using this exercise, grab your exercise bar and pull it down to reach your chest. Ensure it remains elevated. Focus on keeping the shoulder girdle in a low position. This will enhance emphasis on lats instead of your biceps.

Pros

- Useful for those unable to finish a pullup properly.
- Availability of flexibility for performing drop sets or reducing/adding more weight.
- Squeezes and engages the lats more effectively, ensuring development of stronger muscles.

Cons

- A kit is required for executing a proper latpulldown.
- Improper execution may result in injury.

- Support and core muscles may not be engaged adequately enough.
- Pull-ups are a far better alternative for those capable of executing them properly.

Smith Press Machine

If you are new to gym exercise regimens, the Smith Press Machine can be an excellent base to start operations. Shrugs, shoulder presses, and rows are easily done when you use this machine.

The barbells can move vertically up or down as well and can go forward or backward as well.

However, when used for bench presses, you must avoid using it while deadlifting or squatting.

Free weights can often be a better alternative. However, this is highly recommended for gym amateurs.

Pros

- Allows you to undergo isolated workouts, therefore targeting each muscle system with a high range of efficiency.
- Weights can be locked out at any moment of time, therefore ensuring maximum safety and reducing the need for an observer.

Cons

- Stabilizer muscle groups are not adequately trained via this equipment.
- The plane of motion while using the equipment can be quite awkward, thus causing less-than-optimal body development at times.

Seated Rowing Machines

Rowing machines are awesome devices, as they focus on toning upper body muscles properly. They are extremely helpful for weight-loss measures since they are an effective and low-impact form of workouts. Based on one's body's weight, they may allow you to burn 700+ calories per hour, provided you exercise vigorously, without giving up.

However, mastering rowing machines can consume quite a bit of time, as one becomes familiar with the motions. It may also exacerbate existing physical issues or injuries that can do a lot more damage in the long run.

Let's take a look at the list of pros and cons:

Pros

- Since the workout does not take a toll on your joints, you may be spared of pains and a general sense of weariness.

Cons

- Those unable to engage arm, leg and core muscle may require special adaptations to use rowing machines effectively.

- Learning how to operate a rowing machine at peak capacity requires time and regular practice.
- Those with limited time with no patience to learn proper techniques are better off working out with other gym equipment.

Resistance Bands

These are exercise equipments that possess several benefits. These are rubbery and short bands that need certain force amounts to be applied in order for proper stretching. They also come with handles attached for each end, allowing you to form loops around trees or pull up bars.

You can even perform squats, rows, bicep curls and a plethora of several other exercises as well. Due to their versatility, you can use them in place of ordinary gym equipment and carry out most gym training sessions with ease.

However, it is vital to note that exercising with them is no mean feat. Some resistance bands can provide over 300 pounds of resistance. When you add in the excess resistance obtained from looping them, it only goes up from there.

Pros

- Perfect for training your core muscles as they target every muscle group in your body in a single go.
- Active engagement of all muscle groups leads to manifold advantages compared to an isolated muscle group workout.
- Improves posture and form due to the limited range of motion, after you've customized it to your requirements.
- Inculcates discipline, leading to a balanced growth of muscle groups and avoids injuries.
- Resistance bands protect your joints well.
- Those recovering from injuries or attempting to rest from hectic workout schedules may find this to be useful.

Cons

- Not recommended if you are looking to develop a professional bodybuilder's physique.
- While better than most gym workouts, resistance training is no match for the most advanced gym equipment for pros.
- Calculation of accurate resistances can be a tricky affair since it depends on several factors.

Foam Rollers

Foam rollers are used as an after workout method, intended for pain relief and so on. They target specific trigger points, which enable them to release built-up stress and pain. Tight and sore areas, pains and aches in several parts of your body can be overcome by utilizing foam rollers. It increases your range of motion, energy levels, reduces the tension that's been built up due to intense exercise and enhances your overall workout recovery rate.

It is even capable of fixing up DOMS symptoms, a dreaded condition that occurs to most people who've just undergone a grueling session. It is worth noting that it is recommended by experts as well as a recovery method.

Areas that are most commonly stressed upon while using foam rollers are hip flexors, IT bands, shoulder blades, hamstrings, quadriceps, glutes, and back.

Many people may benefit from using the foam roller. It doesn't have to be only sportspersons or professionals who derive maximum benefits.

Pros

- Improves your range of motion
- Enhances overall body flexibility
- Quite easy to utilize it
- Rather than turning to costly massages, this serves as a much more effective and cheaper option.
- It has been shown to prevent the occurrence of post-workout injuries.

- Aids the body's performance in workout sessions.
- It enables faster muscle recovery periods.
- Sore and tight muscles can be stretched and released for better relief.

Cons

- Excessive pressure could again hurt your chances of recovering quickly.
- Benefits may not be visible immediately after you use the foam roller. It takes some time to work out well.
- Those who have no experience in using this should prefer to stay away since improper usage can cause additional injuries.

Stretching Exercises to Master

Stretching matters! Stretching before (warm-up) and after the workout is important in many contexts. If you are stretching, make sure you are stretching on schedule. Here is why warm-up stretching is key to your proper workout.

- It prepares your body for the exercises.
- Stretching eliminates the stiffness and provides the needed flexibility and motion.
- It helps in reducing the possibilities of injuries during exercising

- Warm up stretches help in knowing your body and increases blood circulation
- You can reduce the chances of muscle soreness and muscle strain by performing warm-up stretching
- It also helps you in getting relief from pain during menstruation cycle.
- It increases the overall effectiveness of exercising

Importance of Stretching after Exercising

Stretching after the exercise is equally important due to the following reasons:

- Increases flexibility

Performing post-workout stretching makes your body well-toned and enables you to perform exercises with much ease. Stretching after workout releases the stiffness from your muscles such that next time when you perform exercises, they would be more flexible and at a comfortable state.

- Stops the production of lactic acid

To stop the production of lactic acid after muscle workout, stretching is beneficial. As the muscles produce lactic acid, the muscles become sore and fatigued. Stretching after exercising eliminates such a situation from arising.

- Boosts energy

If you want to stay energized even after a workout session, stretching is what you need to perform. When you stretch properly, you will feel no loss of energy. It helps the body to cool down after the workout session. It makes the body to release endorphins which adds an overall giddy feeling in your body.

- Relieves mental stress

Stretching is not only for muscles but also for a healthy mind. It keeps your mind in the state of tranquility, calm and serene.

Types of Stretching

Now that we know the importance of stretching, let's focus on the various stretching types that you can effortlessly perform.

Spinal twist

This stretching is beneficial for the lower back. To perform it, follow these steps:

- Lie flat with your hand outstretched
- Lift one of your legs and lay it across the second such that your knee is touching the thigh of another leg.
- Shoulders should touch the ground
- The other leg should be kept straight
- Hold the stretch and repeat it with another leg

Upper back stretch

Upper back stretch can be done in multiple ways. These include:

- By performing a rounded back stretch by stretching your hand and shoulder forward.
- By flexing your neck up and down
- By performing lateral neck flexions. To do this, keep your head straight with chin up. Now tilt your neck to one side such that your chin is always up. Repeat with the other side.
- By performing cobra pose
- By lowering your back using an exercise ball

Shoulder stretch

This can be done either by performing overhead shoulder stretch, posterior shoulder stretch or shoulder flexion stretch or simply by squeezing your shoulders.

- You can squeeze your shoulders by resting your shoulders in an upright position then slowly trying to push them towards each other.
- Overhead shoulder stretch is performed by lifting one of your arms overhead and then bending the elbow. Now place your other hand to the outer side of the elbow and push elbow in the interior side.
- Posterior shoulder stretch is performed by laying your hand across your chest, parallel to the floor. Now with the other

hand try to push your elbow in towards your chest.

Downward dog

This stretch is beneficial for hamstring and calves stretching.

- To perform this place your body in an inverted V position such that your toes are pointed towards the front of the mat.

Hamstring stretch

Hamstring stretch can be performed by standing, sitting or by laying on your back.

- Standing hamstring involves placing your leg over a box or flat surface the height of which is approximately your knee height. The hips should be facing forward. Keep the leg straight and slowly try to bend forward keeping the hips and back straight. Hold and repeat with the other leg.
- Sitting hamstring is done by sitting on the floor such that one of your legs is stretched outward and another leg is bent and in resting position. Now try to bring your hand to your feet such that your chest touches your thigh.

Foam Rolling

Besides stretching, what's trending these days in big gyms is foam rolling. It works by reducing the muscle tension and increasing the blood flow in the area you want. Some of the types of foam rolling involve:

- Calf roll

Sit on the floor with your legs outstretched in front. Place the foam roll under your ankles. Place your hands on the floor behind your hip. Slowly lift your hip up putting your body weight on to your hands. Roll the foam roller up and down your calf muscles.

- Glutesroll

Glutes form roll is done by sitting on top of the form roll with one of the leg outstretched in front and other in an upright bent position. Place your hand behind for support and begin rolling.

- Lower backroll

The lowerback foam roll is performed by placing the foam roller beneath your lower back. Sit with the support of the foam roller. Place your leg in 90-degree position resting on the floor. Start rolling up and down with the support of foam roll.

- Lats roll

Lie on one of your sides and place the roll under your armpit horizontally. The hand under which the roll is put should be outstretched and resting on your floor while the other should be in front. Roll your body over the foam such that it travels to your lat till the bottom of the ribcage.

- Groin roll

Lie upside down on the floor and place the foam roller horizontally beneath one side of your lower body and lift the leg outside. Roll on the foam roll such that it travels to the thigh by simultaneously rotating your leg outward.

Foam rolling is much easier to do. Both stretching and foam rolling have their benefits. Performing stretches after foam rolling before and after exercises is recommended.

Weight Loss Program

I have designed the program painstakingly by keeping the energy requirements, muscle training, and other factors in mind. I have ensured that you hit each muscle group at least once during the week(or during the training period).

So, a possible combination could be this:

Day 1: Exercises for legs/glutes

Day 2: Exercises for chest/triceps

Day 3: Exercises for back/biceps

Day 4: Exercises for shoulders/abs

Day 5: Plyometrics

Day 6: Rest (no exercise, just rest)

Day 1: Exercises for Legs/Glutes

1. Single-Leg Deadlift

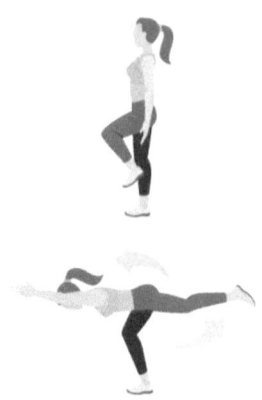

This exercise works wonders for the balance and stability of your body. You do feel the burns in your back and lower body initially, but over time it becomes a part of your routine. Single leg deadlifts can work wonders when they are combined with lunges, hip-thrusts, or any other single-leg dormant exercise.

Benefits

- All the major muscles including thighs, hamstrings, gluteus maximus, gluteus medius, ankles, and the core are worked up.
- You burn fat faster.

- You gain the balance on your body.
- It is a helpful way to build your buttock area.
- This exercise also enhances your nervous system.

Steps to Follow

- Stand erect with both feet closed and in alignment with the hips.
- Shift your body weight to your left leg and bend your left knee softly.
- Straighten your right arm forward to make a ninety-degree angle with your right leg.
- Now slowly take your right leg backward and bend your back to make your right palm touch your feet.
- The right leg should be parallel to the floor once you have taken it backward, your back should be erect and arm should be at 90-degree angle.
- At the end of your position, your head and tip of your right feet should be in one line and parallel to the ground.
- Come back in the reverse order to your original standing position. Now do this with another leg. This would be one rep.

Reps

Begin with 3 sets of 10 reps each with no weights. As you gain endurance, add some weights and do 3 sets of 25 reps each.

2. Lateral Lunge

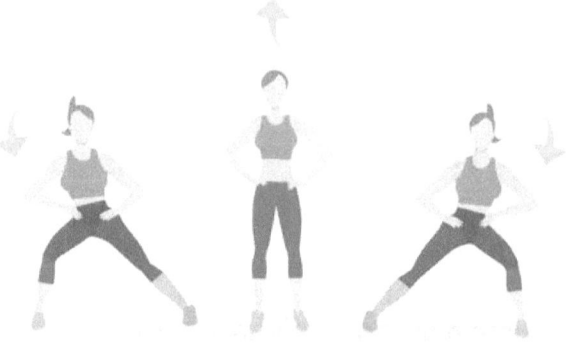

When you have a busy schedule, you wish to gain the maximum out of whatever time you get to work out. Therefore, you wish to focus on exercises that focus on not just one area, but rather benefit your stamina and build on the whole. Lateral lunges or side lunges are the best way to achieve this. The more you practice, the stronger you become, and the more active you become.

Benefits

- Your hips become tighter and sharply sculpted.
- Ankles become more mobile and strong.
- This exercise strengthens your inner thighs and glutes.
- The body gets more adaptive to sudden movements and you find it easier to run and walk.

Steps to Follow

- Stand with your feet spread to shoulder width and toes pointed forward.
- Hold your hands together in front of your chest and keep them there throughout the exercise.
- Hold your left foot in place, and take your right foot to the right as wide as possible. You can also use weights to carry from one position to another.
- Land your right foot on the floor while stretching your leg till the left one is straight.
- Take your hips and knees down (like you do in a squat) on the right side, ensuring that your toes are pointing forward the whole time.
- Use your hips to rise and stand at ease.
- Repeat this on the left side, this time stepping out with your left leg. This is one rep.

Reps

Do 10 reps on each side, and complete 3 sets like this.

3. Ice Skater

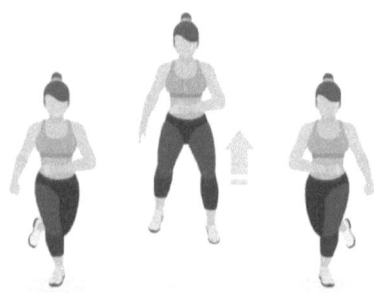

Ice skater exercise not only acts as a great exercise for the leg muscles but it also tones them up. Not only this, ice skater is a great aerobic exercise and boosts your cardiovascular health.

Steps to follow

- Start the process by being in a standing position.
- Keep your hips shoulder-width apart.
- Bend your right knee 90 degrees and position your left leg behind the right leg.
- Keep your left arm across your right leg.
- Position your right arm out to your side.
- One rep will consist of jumping a few feet to the other side and switching your position of arms and legs.

Benefits

This move challenges your balance and tones your outer thighs, butt, lower back, and hips.

Reps

15 reps form one set. Perform 3 sets.

4. Reverse Lunge

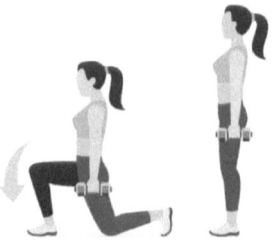

Reverse lunges are an efficient way to get your body into motion. This exercise is great for your lower body and a total body tune-up. Moving a single leg increases your balance, stability and sculpts your leg, which helps in carrying those high heels with confidence. It is probably the best single-leg work out that you can do. To fetch better results, you can also use weights.

Benefits

- In the beginning, your entire backside is strengthened and toned, because your quads, glutes, and hamstrings are targeted while doing the exercise.
- It improves the running technique as your knee learns to stabilize itself over the toe.
- Reverse lunges improve your mobility and motion, which helps you prevent knee pain and ankle sprains.
- When your body gets used to this exercise, you are able to squat deeper

and perform many other exercises easily.

- It also lowers your back pain.

Steps to Follow

- Take an erect position with your feet slightly apart in alignment with your shoulders.
- Pick up your right leg and step back keeping your left leg in place.
- Lower your right leg while taking it back, and land on fingers of your right toe with heels facing up.
- Make your right knee touch the ground making an angle of 90 degrees between your right thigh and left calf.
- Now slowly push through the heel of your left leg to return to the standing position.
- Repeat with taking your left leg backward. This is one rep.

Reps

Do 8-10 reps on one leg and then 8-10 on the other. Do 3 sets of such repetitions in total.

Day 2: Exercises for Chest/Triceps

1. Bench Press

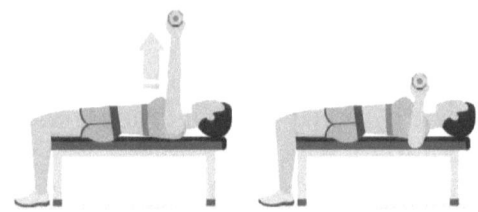

Do not get swayed away with all the misconceptions that discourage you from performing bench press exercise. This is perhaps because bench presses at the local gym are dominated by men. Further, a lot of women believe that this exercise will shrink their breast-size. Believe me, nothing like this is ever going to happen if you do the exercise right!

Beat the stereotypes and go ahead with it, also because it is one of the most effective chest exercises which helps you in working on several muscle groups at once and also helps you in firming up your pecs.

Benefits

- Bench press keeps your breasts in shape and prevents them from sagging.
- It improves your posture, thus enhancing your confidence.
- The bench press is as much an upper body workout as it is a lower body

workout. All in all, it strengthens your body.

- It also improves your flexibility and tones your body perfectly.

Steps to follow

- Lie on the bench.
- Hold the dumbbells with a medium grip without pressurizing your hand. Keep your thumbs around the bar.
- Strengthen your arms and unrack the dumbbells.
- Next, push the dumbbellsto a lower level towards your mid-chest.
- Press the dumbbellsback to the normal position until your arms are straight.

Reps

Start with a set of 5 reps.

2. Pushup

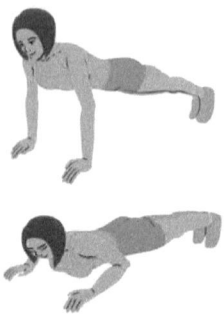

If you want to strengthen your forearms, the biceps, and triceps, there could be no better and easier exercise than push-ups. The best part of pushups is that they can be performed right at your home without you needing to hit a gym.

Benefits

- Pushups help women by strengthening their chest and toning their arms.
- They stabilize and balance your body by working on your muscles.
- Pushups help you in toning your legs and buttocks by making them grow stronger and leaner.

Steps to follow

- To begin with, get yourself into a plank position.
- Keep your hands slightly outside the level of your shoulders.

- Next, lower your body gradually till your chest touches the floor. Make sure that when you lower yourself, your elbows are tucked such that your upper arms make an angle of 45-degree with your torso.
- Regain your original plank position.

Reps

You should do 16-20 pushups per day.

3. Pull Over

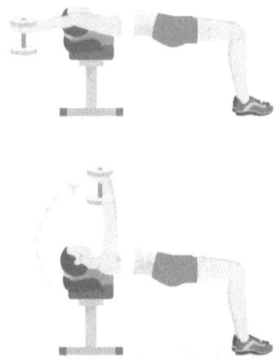

If you think that your little girls need some lifting, dumbbell pullovers might just be an ideal pick for you. This exercise works on your pectoral muscles which are located close to the breasts. This way, this exercise, works by enhancing and beautifying your bust line and lifting your breasts. To get the best results, it is highly recommended to perform the exercise in the right way and your little girls will be back in their shape in no time.

Benefits

- Dumbbell pullover can help you in enhancing the shape of your breasts and lifting them up.
- In addition to working on your chest, it also tones your triceps and lats.

Steps to follow

- Start the process by lying on a bench.
- Hold a dumbbell in your hand.
- Ensure that your feet are placed flat on the floor and your knees are bent.
- Protect your lower back from any pressure by tightening your abdominals.
- Next, extend your arms and raise the dumbbell directly over your face.
- Extend your arms fully such that your palms face the ceiling and the weights hang vertically.
- Next, bend your elbow and bring your arms back to their normal position with an arc-like motion.

Reps

15-20 reps per day

4. Pec deck Machine

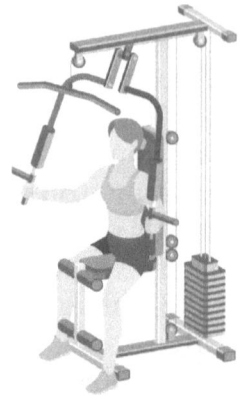

Pec deck machine also called as machine fly exercise is based on the free weight chest fly. The exercise tones up your pectoralis major muscles, shoulders, and the rib cage. You don't need to believe that since you have breasts, pec training is not needed. It is needed, and rightly so, because of an array of benefits that it offers.

Benefits

- Pec deck machine can help you in improving your posture by working on one of the largest muscles in the body.
- With the improved posture, comes enhanced looks and boosted confidence.
- This exercise will open up your chest, thus helping you in breathing easier.
- If you want to augment your breasts, pec deck machine is one exercise that you need to try.

Steps to Follow

- Position yourself on the pec deck machine comfortably.
- Almost all machines have an adjustable seat pad that can be lifted or lowered. Make necessary arrangements to ensure that you are seated comfortably with your feet on the floor and the spine supported by the back pad.
- Extend your arms while grabbing the handles of the machine and ensuring that your wrists and elbows are in line with your shoulder.
- Choose a weight setting. Start with smaller weights you feel comfortable with.
- Press the arms together in front of your chest with a controlled movement.
- Once the arms are closed fully, pause for a second and bring your arm back to the original position.

Reps

3 sets of 10 to 12 reps

Day 3: Exercises for Back/Biceps

1. Biceps curl

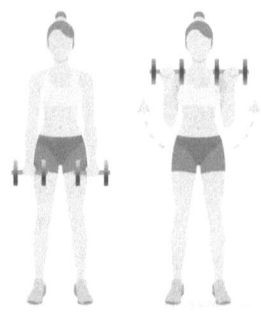

Having strong biceps is important, not just for beauty purposes but for your overall well-being as well. This is because you use them every time you bend your elbow and this is why you must keep them in top-notch condition.

Steps to follow

- Biceps curl can be done in two ways – when you are standing or sitting on a bench.
- If you want to challenge yourself truly, I will highly recommend you to perform them standing.
- You might want to perform a single arm curl or curl both arms at once depending on your end goal.
- Curl both the arms if you want to earn shoulder stability, however, if you simply want to do strength training, curl alternate arms.

- Hold a pair of dumbbells with your palms positioned forward.
- Bend your elbow and pull your hand towards your shoulder with control.
- Keep your wrist and upper arm still.
- Pause for a second and regain your original position.

Reps

Ideally, choose a weight which will let you perform three sets of 8-12 reps.

2. One Arm Dumbbell

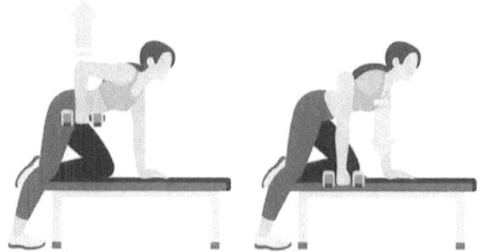

If you want to strengthen your back, one arm dumbbell ticks all the right boxes. Although a bit challenging move, this exercise will strengthen your core, arms, and shoulders all at once.

Benefits

- It strengthens your back along with upper arms, shoulder, and core.
- Enhances the blood flow and/, in turn, burns calories on the go.
- Your coordination, agility, and balance will improve.

Steps to follow

- Position yourself on a bench by resting one leg on the floor and the other on the bench.
- Hold a 10-pound dumbbell in your right hand. Keep your other hand on your back and slowly bend your knees and hips and lower your torso until it is parallel to the floor.

- Keep holding the dumbbell at arm's length.
- Next, pull the dumbbell to the side of the torso without disturbing your position.
- Ensure that your elbow is tucked close to the side. Pause and regain your original position.

Suggested reps

Complete 8 to 12 reps

3. Lat pull down

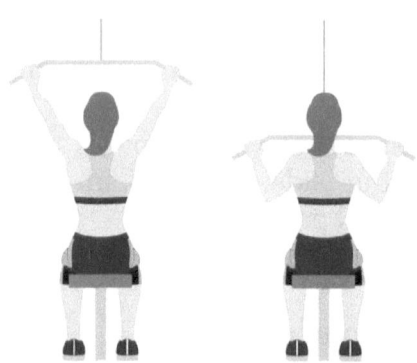

This pull down exercise works on your lats or latissimus dorsi. This is an important muscle which is positioned under the armpits and spreads across the down and back. The best part of exercising this muscle separately is that you are not tiring your triceps and biceps during the process.

Benefits

- Lats pull down tones up your lats muscle.
- It helps you improve your posture so that you can perform pulling movements at ease like using a lawnmower, opening a door and so on.

Steps to follow

- Sit down on the pulldown seat comfortably such that your feet touch the floor.

- Adjust the height of the bar to your seat height. Take the help of a gym trainer in this
- The bar should be positioned such that you can conveniently grab it with your arms without needing to stand up.
- Pull the bar down until it is at a level of your chin.
- Exhale as you pull the bar down.
- Once it is at its bottom position, make the bar return to its original position slowly and gradually while controlling its gradual ascent.

Reps

Perform 8-12 reps in a set.

4. Overhead Shoulder Press

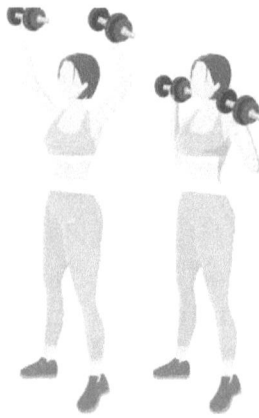

Overhead shoulder press is an amazing exercise which can help you in building your back. If you perform it in a standing position, it can help you work out almost all the major muscles of the upper body including triceps, pectorals, triceps, and trapezius.

Benefits

- It enhances the strength and size of the shoulder muscles, triceps muscles, and trapezius muscles.
- It adds strength to the core muscles.
- It helps you in performing other exercises like the bench press effectively.

Steps to follow

- Graba dumbbell in each hand and position both your hands above your shoulders.

- Make sure that your palms face inside.
- Straighten your arms above you.
- Slightly bend your elbows and regain your original position. This will complete one rep.

Suggested reps

Perform 10 reps in total.

Day 4: Exercises for Shoulders/Abs

1. Seated Dumbbell Press

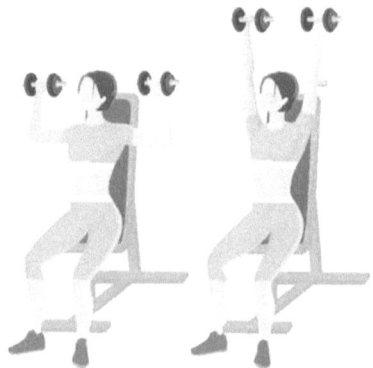

One of the best ways to obtain strong shoulders is by performing seated dumbbell press. The exercise works on your shoulders improves their strength and enhances your body's overall ability.

Benefits

- It helps you get sexier and toned shoulders.
- Improves the strength of shoulders, and enhances your balance.

Steps to follow

- Sit in a comfortable position on a utility bench or press bench with a back support.

- Hold the dumbbells at your ear-level and place them lengthwise.
- Straighten your arms without locking your elbow.
- Push the dumbbells up as you exhale.
- Pause for a second and let them come to their original position as you inhale. This will complete one rep.

Suggested reps

Do 3 sets of 15 reps each and increase the weights as your body gets used to them.

2. Pike push up

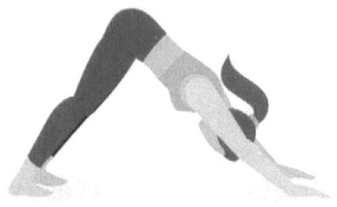

This list of shoulder training exercises cannot be completed without mentioning the pike pushup. This is a slightly different version of the conventional push up exercise and indeed a little more difficult. The exercise works on your shoulder muscles and provides them with the required strength.

Benefits

- Pike pushups guarantee you extreme flexibility in your body
- This exercise helps women build shoulder strength
- Pike pushups help increase the muscle mass of your arms
- This exercise helps you reach the ideal headstand push up posture

Steps to follow

- Firstly, warm up the body in order to get it ready for the pushups. Some light stretching would help.
- Get yourself in the traditional push up posture.

- Lift your body up such that the legs are moving towards the body.
- Get into the correct posture when your body is able to hold on to the V shape.
- Bend your elbows sideways till the head touches the ground.
- A higher intensity workout would involve you lifting your leg in the air as your body goes down.

Suggested Reps

Essentially, the pike push up exercise can be performed by women in sets of 10 to 15 per day.

3. Elbow plank

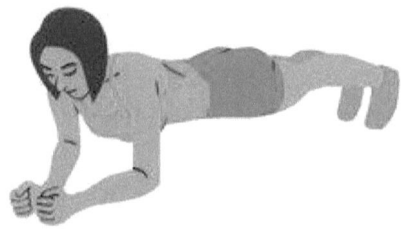

We are all aware of the fact that the best way to make abs is through planks. Talking about elbow plank, it is a more difficult version of the plank exercise. However, it provides better results and helps in increasing strength. It is the best way to acquire toned abs without engaging in crunches.

Benefits

- Elbow planks are the best form of exercise if you are targeting a full body workout.
- Regular planks can actually lead to a toned belly.
- This sort of exercise can also reduce back pain.
- The body's flexibility is greatly improved with the help of elbow planks.

Steps to follow

- Firstly, rest on the floor, lifting the body off the ground. Help the body rest on the forearms placed on the floor.

- Raise your body off the floor while shifting the balance from the knees to the toes
- In this position, contract the abdominal muscles.
- The back should remain flat throughout the exercise.
- Repeat.

Suggested reps

This posture of the elbow planks could be held for about 20 to 30 seconds initially, increase the time period of 60 seconds gradually. This set if repeated three times.

Day 5: Plyometrics

1. Jump squats

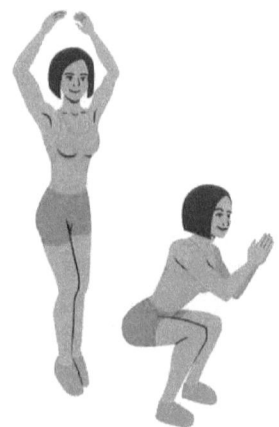

If you are looking for a toned body, jump squats are the ideal way to go. These essentially work on the quads and the calves to increase the body's strength in the lower back, thighs, and legs. There are different kinds of jump squats that cater to different body types.

Benefits

- Weight loss is one of the most direct benefits of jump squats.
- It adds shape to your thighs and legs.
- Jump squats are also useful for strengthening the lower back in women.
- This workout helps improve the cardio-respiratory system.

- Jump squats can also condition the body by increasing the heart rate during the work out phase.

Steps

- First and foremost, bring your body to the squat position. This means, bend your knees and attain a sitting posture, with the thighs parallel to the floor. You could hold on to this posture.
- Gradually release your body upwards and raise your hands above your head
- As you jump, try to get back in the original position with the hands and legs placed as before

Suggested reps

You can execute 3 sets of 15 repetitions.

2. Frog jump

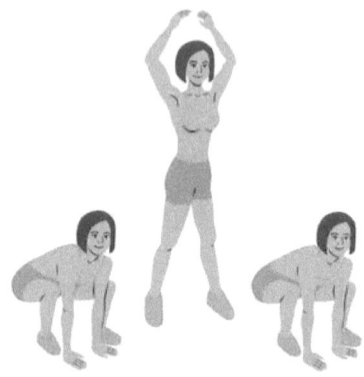

Frog jumping is a rather interesting exercise to gain muscle mass and improve its strength. In fact, in many situations, this is practiced as a sport or as a competitive event instead of just a workout. This plyometric exercise actually helps you maintain your cardio fitness by pumping up the heart rate. As the name suggests, this exercise requires you to jump up like a frog.

Benefits

- The calves, hamstring and the leg muscles are strengthened with the help of frog jumps
- It releases the pain points in the legs and makes them more flexible
- This workout caters to the stubborn fat accumulation in the body and releases them
- It also helps boost your memory

Steps to follow

- Start by maintaining a standing position and keeping your legs at shoulder width
- Lower your body to a squat position, in a 3/4th sitting posture
- Hold that position for a couple of seconds and then jump up aggressively to land up 2 feet in front of you
- Restart the exercise from this position again

Suggested reps

Once you have mastered the technique, you could either practice it in sets of 10 or 15 or you could also just perform the workout for 30 seconds

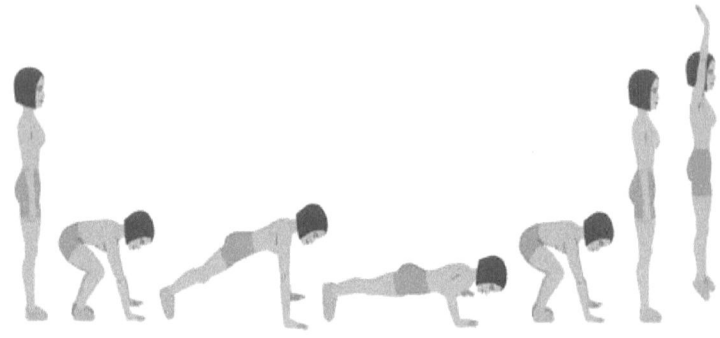

3. Burpees

Burpees or squat thrust is one of the most effective exercises that target the entire body at one go. This aerobic exercise is actually carried out in four different steps.

Benefits

- Firstly, the burpees is a full body exercise that aims to work on every single muscle in the body
- It works on cardiovascular fitness by monitoring the breathing process and the heart rate
- It aims to increase the muscular strength and mobility in the body
- You could combine this exercise with other workouts to derive the best out of it

Steps to follow

- Initially, start with the standing posture and drop down to a squat posture
- The hands should stay in front of your feet on the floor
- Kick your feet towards the back such that you maintain a raised plank position
- Round this process up by releasing your posture and leaping into the air with your arms above your body

Suggested reps

Initially, you could start off with 20 or 25 burpees to be completed in a minute. You could gradually increase your stamina to reach about 100 reps to be completed in about 15 minutes.

Conclusion

This brings us to the end of this book. I hope this book must have inspired you throughout, and helped you in your weight loss journey.

As is evident, smallest life choices matter. From when you eat to what you eat and how you eat; from when you sleep to how much you sleep; from how you exercise to what kinds of equipment you use – everything matters!

Thus, it is essential to ensure that you are making healthy life choices, and taking out enough time for yourself.

I hope this book helped you in your goal of leading a healthier lifestyle and losing weight.

Thanks for reading. If you liked the book, do not forget to share it with your friends and family. Also, don't forget to leave a review on the Amazon page!

www.amazon.com/dp/B07WCZW125

www.ingramcontent.com/pod-product-compliance
Lightning Source LLC
Chambersburg PA
CBHW061259280526
45784CB00002B/815